John C. Thorowgood

Notes on asthma

Its nature, forms, and treatment

John C. Thorowgood

Notes on asthma
Its nature, forms, and treatment

ISBN/EAN: 9783742826893

Manufactured in Europe, USA, Canada, Australia, Japa

Cover: Foto ©Lupo / pixelio.de

Manufactured and distributed by brebook publishing software
(www.brebook.com)

John C. Thorowgood

Notes on asthma

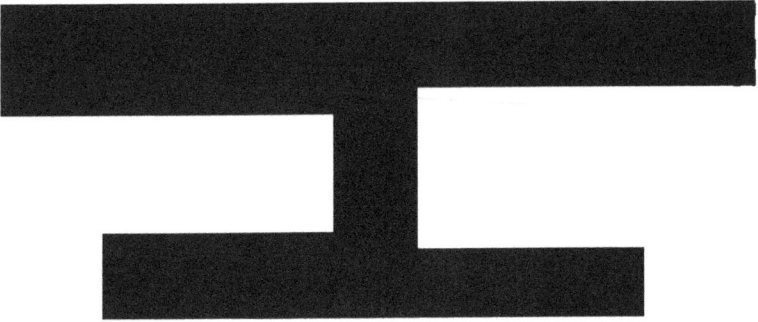

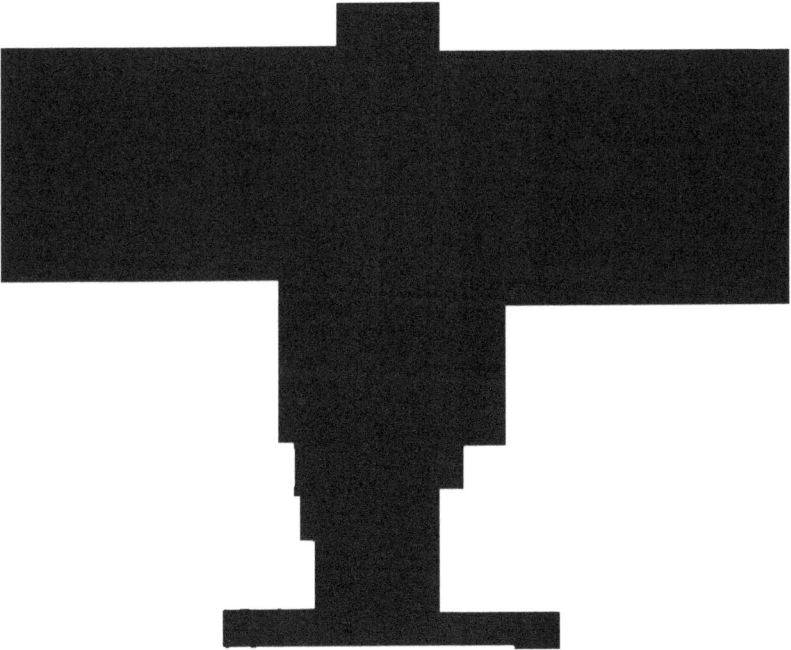

PREFACE TO SECOND EDITION.

THE reader of this book must bear in mind that it does not profess to be a systematic Treatise on Asthma. With such a work our Profession has been already well supplied from the pen of the late Dr. HYDE SALTER; and though, since the publication of the first edition of these "Notes," that excellent and talented physician has been called away by death, yet his admirable monograph on Asthma remains to us a valuable embodiment of rich experience and a worthy memorial of the author.

The present work is based upon such notes of Asthma, its forms and complications, as the author has been able to make during his ten years' service as Assistant-Physician to the Victoria-Park Hospital for Diseases of the Chest.

From the cases selected all instances of dyspnœa due to organic heart disease, and all cases of chronic bronchitis with no marked complications in the way of spasmodic or paralytic dyspnœa, are excluded.

The cases recorded range themselves in two divisions, the first comprising instances of pure inorganic spasmodic asthma, due to constitutional and hereditary diathesis, or to individual susceptibility to some specific exciting cause; and among these the purely nervous form of asthma can be well studied.

In the second larger division may be placed instances of complicated and organic asthma; that is to say, asthma, in the sense of a spasmodic or paralytic neurosis, engrafted upon such pulmonary diseases as chronic bronchitis, emphysema of the lungs, or a complication of both these maladies.

Investigation with the laryngoscope having within the last few years materially advanced our knowledge of certain troublesome and dangerous forms of dyspnœa, I have in this edition introduced a short chapter (X.) containing some practical remarks on the diagnosis of laryngeal and tracheal dyspnœa.

For purposes of treatment it is of some consequence to distinguish spasmodic asthma, due to contraction of the small bronchial tubes, from dyspnœa due to bronchial and pulmonary paralysis; pathologically, however, these two conditions are not very distinct, for the paralytic state of lung is often a consequence of repeated spasmodic seizures in the first instance.

I believe the connection of spasm with paralysis is far closer than some may think; just as states of hyperæsthesia and anæsthesia — widely separate symptomatically — may not differ so much in their essential causation.

With these views I have insisted much on the value of nerve tonics as curative agents in asthma; sedatives and antispasmodics at intervals, and on emergencies, not being incompatible with tonics as our really curative medicines.

The prolonged use of expectorants is to be strongly reprobated; founded often on error in mistaking purely nervous for inflammatory symptoms, it is a practice likely to exhaust and enfeeble the bronchial muscle, to injure the tone of the digestive organs, and thus to do immense mischief.

Another thing that I would enter a caution against in the treatment of asthma, is "poly-pharmacy," especially when using drugs from which we expect definite and specific action, such as strychnine, belladonna, arsenic, ipeca-cuanha, or quinia. I cannot, myself, with any sort of faith combine belladonna with strych-nine, or either of these with opium or morphia; and I believe that one result of our advancing diagnostic skill will be to simplify our phar-macy and make our cures more certain and more lasting.

JOHN C. THOROWGOOD.

61 WELBECK STREET, CAVENDISH SQUARE, W.,
January, 1873.

CONTENTS.

ON ASTHMA.

CHAPTER I.

Spasmodic Asthma.—The disease presents marked symptoms during life, yet has no morbid anatomy.—Action of the thoracic and bronchial muscles in respiration.—Asthma a spasm of the small muscles encircling the air-tubes of the lung, resembling gastric or intestinal spasm.—Varieties of Asthma. —Hæmic Asthma due to circulation of disordered or diseased blood.—Reflex Asthma from nervous excitement or irritation.—Specific Asthma caused by various animal or vegetable emanations.—Complicated and Organic Asthma distinct from the above, and to be treated of separately.

ONE who is in the grasp of a fit of true spasmodic asthma always presents an abundance of symptoms, which, while they last, are distressing enough to endure or to witness; and yet, when things seem to be about at the worst, and the patient well-nigh at his last gasp, a remission comes on, the spasm yields, air enters the lungs, and the attack subsides, coincidently often with access of cough and mucous expectoration.

During the intervals between his attacks the patient probably enjoys fair health, and, as a general rule, lives to a good age; at last, he, like the rest of mankind, dies; and after death what do we find as the morbid anatomy to explain the well-marked symptoms seen during life?

This question may be answered in the words of Sir T. Watson, as true now as when he first uttered them years ago in his lectures,--" The bodies of asthmatics have often, on being examined after death, presented no vestige whatever of disease, either in the lungs or in the heart; evidence that the phenomena attending a fit of asthma may be the result of pure spasm."

So, too, the late Dr. Hyde Salter, in his classical treatise on Asthma, says: "A man may have been known during his life to have had attacks of asthma, he may have seemed over and over again almost *in articulo mortis* from want of breath; and yet, if death from some ther cause gives an opportunity of examining is lungs, they may be found apparently in very way healthy—no trace of inflammation r its products, the vesicular structure perfectly ormal, the passages leading to it lined by a calthy and unchanged membrane, the cavities f the pleura free from all abnormal contents, heir surfaces smooth and apposed, the heart ound. The disease shows no cause, and has eft no trace either in the respiratory or circu- atory systems — in fact, no trace anywhere. Where then shall we locate it ? What is its tarting-point ? We may, I think, lay it down s a rule that all those diseases that leave no rganic trace of their existence produce their ymptoms through the nervous system."—*Page* o, *2nd Edition.*

While we may consider it proved possible or a person to have violent attacks of spas- nodic asthma without there being present any tructural changes in the lungs; yet, after a while, the serious perversion of lung function aused by the repetition of the fits cannot but ead to some amount of structural change,

and the microscope will probably show some
granular or fatty degeneration in the air cells
of the lung, though to the naked eye appearances may be normal.

Since, then, morbid anatomy tells us but
little in cases of true spasmodic asthma, we
must seek our knowledge from the teachings
of physiology, and from the observed phenomena of the asthmatic paroxysm, seeing that
our present purpose is entirely with spasmodic
asthma, presumed to be uncomplicated with
any detectable lesion of lungs, heart, or any
other organ.

The essence of a fit of spasmodic asthma
consists in tonic spasm of the bronchial muscles;
these bronchial muscles being the unstriped
contractile fibres which encircle the air-tubes
of the lungs, just as the muscular fibres of the
intestines surround those tubes with a contractile force.

The larger bronchial tubes have their cartilaginous rings as elastic spring openers; the
smaller tubes, lying nearest to the vesicular
parts of the lung, have no cartilaginous rings.

but are entirely muscular; and Laennec and Reisseissen, and more recently Gratiolet, have detected muscular fibres in air-tubes less than one line in transverse diameter. The contractility of these fibres under the influence of electrical, chemical, and mechanical stimuli was demonstrated in a series of ingenious and conclusive experiments by Dr. Williams many years ago. When speaking of the effect of certain remedies in asthma, I shall have occasion to refer again to those experiments.

The muscularity of the smallest bronchia has been recently demonstrated by Prof. Rindfleisch. This observer finds that these small circular fibres form a sort of sphincter where the bronchia are continuous with the infundibula.

The fibres are capable of much elongation, and rest upon a very close-meshed plexus of capillaries, which resemble the pulmonary vascular plexus.

In brown induration of the lung these muscular bands become hypertrophied.

Paul Bert, Traube, and others, have demon-

strated how the respiration can be arrested by
irritation of the pneumogastric or laryngeal
nerves, or those supplying the Schneiderian
mucous membrane of the nose.

The arrest is much more easily obtained
during expiration than inspiration.

It has been shown by MM. Valentin and
Volkman that irritation of the pneumogastric
or vagus nerve will cause contraction of the
air-tubes and approximation of the ends of
their cartilaginous rings, and this fact of the
lungs contracting under the influence of the
vagi nerves has been confirmed by the experiments of Traube and Bernard. These matters
have important bearing on the causes and
phenomena of the asthmatic fit, as well as on
the therapeutic means we employ to relieve
the same.

The precise function of the bronchial muscles in the mechanism of respiration appears
to be a matter of dispute with various observers,
and this uncertainty has led to more than
one theory in explanation of the asthmatic
paroxysm.

In ordinary expiration the bronchial muscles contract rhythmically by virtue of the resilience imparted to them by their own natural elasticity; by this action they quicken the expulsion of foul air from the lung cells, and accommodate the size of the tubes to the lessening bulk of the lung.

In spasmodic asthma extreme expiration, as in a fit of coughing or laughing, often brings on the paroxysm; a fact interesting in connexion with the observation just referred to, that arrest of respiration by irritation of nerve is more easily obtained in expiration than during inspiration.

It seems probable that under abnormal circumstances the bronchial muscles can act during either inspiration or expiration. They act with irregular vehemence in cough; with clonic spasm in whooping-cough; with tonic spasm in asthma.

These views accord in the main with those of Haller, Reisseissen, Radclyffe Hall, Elliotson, Williams, and Brown-Séquard; and I believe will, with perhaps some modifications, become established under increasing observation and experience.

Dr. Von Bamberger (*a*) lays much stress on spasm of the diaphragm as "the most frequent and the most influential, though not the only cause of spasmodic asthma;" and he alludes to paralysis of the diaphragm as causing asthma in some cases of progressive muscular atrophy observed by Duchenne. These, however, would be cases of what would better be called "paralytic dyspnœa," and are similar to cases of dyspnœa resulting from impaired action of the phrenic nerves.

That the diaphragm is a muscle especially concerned in the respiratory act of inspiration is well known. The fibres of this muscle take origin from the inner surface of the cartilages, and a little of the osseous part of all the ribs which form the margin of the thorax,—that is to say, the five false ribs and the last true one; one narrow muscular slip arises from the xiphoid cartilage, and all these muscular

_____

(*a*) Syd. Soc. "Year-book, 1865-6," p. 140.

fibres curve upwards and inwards to join the central tendon of the diaphragm.

This muscle acts in inspiration by contracting, and as a consequence it descends and becomes an inclined plane, whose direction is downwards and forwards, while the cavity of the thorax is enlarged, and that of the abdomen diminished.

In expiration the diaphragm rises, being pressed up by the contraction of the abdominal muscles, and after a complete expiration its upper surface is on a level with the lower border of the fourth rib.

In the adult male, as is well known, ordinary respiration is chiefly diaphragmatic, the ribs and sternum not moving much. In strong inspiration, the elevation and expansion movements of the thorax are completely developed by such muscles as are connected with the ribs. Thus, the scaleni muscles draw up and fix the first rib; the levatores costarum, extending obliquely downwards and forwards from the transverse processes of the dorsal vertebræ to the margins of the ribs, between their angles and tubercles, also act in raising the ribs from behind.

Between the ribs are the two planes of intercostal muscles, their fibres decussating with each other, the external muscles passing downwards and forwards, the internal downwards and backwards.

The external intercostals act to raise the ribs and push forward the sternum. In drawing up the ribs they slightly rotate the bodies on the pivot joints of the costo-vertebral articulation, and evert the lower borders of those bones ; at the same time the middle and lower intercostal spaces are widened, for the ribs are spread asunder somewhat like those of a fan. This arises from the peculiar mode of attachment of the last rib, which is prevented from ascending with the rest by the manner in which the quadratus lumborum binds it to the ilium, so that it serves to spread or separate them from one another. The internal intercostals, acting by themselves, tend to draw down the ribs, and so aid in expiration.

The elevation of the ribs is further assisted

by the serratus magnus and other muscles connected with the spine and the scapula; and
when the respiratory movement is very for-
cibly performed the scapula itself is drawn up
by the muscles that descend to it from the
neck, and the upper part of the thoracic cavity
is much enlarged.

During the paroxysm of spasmodic asthma
it is well known how the scapulæ are drawn
up and the shoulders raised; while, by fixing
his elbows or arms, the asthmatic gains additional expansive power on the ribs.

The hollow at the epigastrium, and the distress often complained of there, show the effort
the diaphragm is making to expand the chest
below.

Despite all these straining efforts of the
thoracic muscles air cannot be got to enter
the lungs; these organs are spasmodically
fixed, and the small tubes and air cells will
not act in unison with the muscles of inspiration; hence the distressing want of breath, and
hence all the external straining which we be-
hold during a paroxysm of asthma. More ·

or less of air may be imprisoned within the air-cells, but the further interchange of air in the ordinary process of inspiration and expiration is well nigh entirely arrested and at a standstill.

When the arrest is complete, symptoms of asphyxia, with deep lividity of face, come on, as when a person inhales deadly gas ; but when things seem at the very worst the paroxysm yields, possibly in consequence of the carbonic acid accumulated in the blood acting as an anti-spasmodic, so that the extreme danger from asphyxia brings, in fact, relief to the sufferer.

Having thus briefly sketched the nature and mode of production of the asthmatic paroxysm, I do not profess in these "Notes" to enter upon any discussion of the various theories that have been put forth. My purpose is mainly to offer some remarks on the treatment of the different varieties of asthma ; and for a complete history of the complaint, and of all the views that have been put forth concerning it, I must refer my reader to the complete and well-known treatise of Dr. Hyde Salter.

I am myself satisfied to make the distinguishing mark of asthma to be a spasm or cramp seizing on the muscular fibres which encircle the small bronchial tubes, and which we call the bronchial muscles. In asthma these muscles remain spasmodically fixed, and so will not let air in or out of the lungs, though the muscles of the trunk of the body are straining their utmost to expand the chest and promote inspiration.

In some respects asthma is to the lungs what colic is to the bowels, or angina pectoris to the heart; it is in fact a form of muscular cramp, and when we know exactly what muscular cramp is, we shall be a step further in our knowledge of the pathogenesis of asthma.

We know that arrested or disordered circulation of the blood through a muscle may cause cramp in the muscle. In the later stages of cholera, when the blood, drained of its serum, becomes too thick to flow freely through the vessels, severe cramps are apt to come on. In cases, too, of angina pectoris, one of the most constant morbid appearances found after death is degeneration or abnormal arrangement of the coronary arteries which circulate the blood through the muscular substance of the heart.

I am aware that the theory of the asthmatic fit being due to a spasmodic setting, or contraction of the bronchial muscles has been controverted by some; but I could never make any other theory in any way accord with observed facts, neither could my valued friend, the late Dr. Hyde Salter, who had seen more of asthma than anyone probably, and who told me not long before his death that he held as firmly as ever to the theory of lung contraction as best explaining the true nature of ordinary spasmodic asthma.

The fact that in asthma the percussion resonance is at times impaired as the lungs become emptied of air, according to the observations of Dr. Walshe, Dr. Flint, and myself, tends to prove that the lung is itself contracted and devoid, in a measure, of air.

Since a free and regular circulation of the blood must depend, for one condition, on the right composition of this fluid, anything that impairs this normal composition may become a cause of irregular circulation. It has long

been observed that many asthmatics are liable
to be attacked by their complaint some time
not long after a meal, especially if the food
taken should have been of unwholesome kind.
In these cases we can with much reason attribute the attack of asthma to some irritating
matter formed in the blood, which, as it circu-
lates through the fibres of the bronchial muscles throws these into a state of spasm. The
morbid matter of gout, rheumatism, or of any
other diathetic disease circulating in the blood,
may thus cause asthma. To this form of asthma,
arising from the circulation of disordered or
diseased blood, the name of *Hæmic asthma*
has been applied.

In a different class of cases the asthmatic fit
may come on so instantly on the reception of
unwholesome food by the stomach, or on the
application of cold or other irritant to the body,
that we cannot attribute the conveyance of
the irritation to the lungs to the channel of
the blood, and we consider in these cases the
nerves to be the channels through which the
impression is conveyed to the lungs, and bronchial spasm induced. Uterine irritation, a

loaded state of the stomach or bowels, a sudden draught of cold air, or a dash of cold water over the foot, may cause this description of asthma; and it may be described as *Reflex asthma*, since the irritation is reflected from its seat to the lungs through the medium of the nerves.

In another group of cases the cause of the asthmatic paroxysm is found in the air which the patient breathes; this may act as a direct irritant, and provoke spasm in the bronchial tubes, just as undigested food may cause gastric or intestinal spasm; in this class of cases may be placed instances of *Specific asthma*, arising from the smell of hay, or from any special vegetable or animal emanation.

This classification appears to embrace all cases of pure uncomplicated spasmodic asthma, and on it a rational plan of treatment must be based.

Bronchitic, emphysematous, and cardiac asthma stand in another category as instances of complicated or organic asthma, and are treated of in the latter part of this book.

CHAPTER II.

Reasons for viewing spasmodic asthma as a nervous disease.—Dyspnœa sometimes due to paralysis of the bronchial muscles.—Brief description of an ordinary fit of asthma.—Particular varieties of asthma described by Wunderlich and Flint.—Diagnosis of spasmodic asthma from the dyspnœa due to organic brain disease, or to pressure of intra-thoracic tumours.—Affections of the heart and larynx causing dyspnœa and apnœa not to be regarded in the same way as asthma.—Prognosis of asthma usually, but not invariably, favourable.

WE have seen in the foregoing chapter that spasmodic asthma is essentially a nervous disease, due to spasm affecting the muscular fibres which encircle the smaller bronchial tubes.

That asthma, *in the sense of difficulty in the breathing*, may occur from a paralyzed rather than from a spasmodically contracted state of these muscles is a point to be adverted to presently. Usually, but not necessarily, this paralytic dyspnœa is connected with some

C

amount of organic affection of the lung tissue, but that we may have either spasm or paralysis of the bronchial muscle causing asthma, is to me as clear as that we may have spasm or paralysis of the muscular coat of the bladder, leading alike to retention of urine.

In further proof of the nervous nature of asthma we have the suddenness with which the attack comes on, and the absence of premonitory symptoms pointing directly to the lung, such as cough, expectoration, or bronchitis. Nervous excitement will *cause*, and not unfrequently *cure* (page 43), a fit of asthma; and in a rapid way we hear all the sonorous and sibilant wheezings, which have filled the chest during the fit, subside at once into natural respiration as the spasm yields. All these matters attest the nervous nature of the seizure.

The phenomena of the actual asthmatic fit are familiar to most persons. The attack may come on at any period of the twenty-four hours, though commonly it appears towards early morning; its invasion may wake the patient up suddenly from his sleep, or, after waking from a sense of tightness and distress about his chest, the sufferer finds the symptoms increase till he is obliged to sit up, leaning forward, with raised shoulders, bent back, his elbows on his knees, or else his hands grasping some fixed point, the better to enable the muscles of the shoulders to act in expanding the chest.

Much distress is felt at the pit of the stomach, due to the contraction of the diaphragm, and the speech is short, husky, and hardly audible.

The countenance of the asthmatic betokens his distress from want of air; the eyes are prominent, the face red and congested, or else livid and damp, with a cold clammy sweat.

The pulse at the wrist is remarkably small, from the scanty quantity of blood passing through the heart in consequence of the stoppage in the lungs.

The thorax is, as a rule, in a state of extreme distention, and, as a rule, fully resonant on percussion; but at times, in extreme contraction of the lung, percussion resonance is diminished, as has been already stated. On

watching the breathing it is observed to be
difficult, sometimes slow, not more than nine or
ten respirations a minute, at other times very
hurried. Expiration is markedly prolonged,
being often four or five times as long as inspiration. Cough, if present, is short and difficult.
On listening to the chest no healthy breathing can be detected; the chest seems full of
sonorous and sibilant sounds in the air-tubes,
which are constantly changing from one part
of the chest to another; rarely are moist sounds
heard, and the dry sounds just described are
dependent on spasmodic narrowing of the
bronchial tubes, and are not changed by
coughing.

After lasting usually some hours, the attack
subsides, with or without expectoration of
mucus, sometimes frothy, sometimes thick,
and at times in small dark lumps or pellets.
Expectoration is present or absent, according
as the case is one of "humid" or "dry"
asthma. The urine after the attack is turbid
often with lithates, but during the paroxysm
it is watery and pale.

While the description I have thus given of the asthmatic paroxysm will serve as a general one in most cases, it must be remembered that cases may be met with now and then in practice which are true cases of asthma, and yet do not in every particular correspond to the standard descriptions given of that complaint.

Thus Wunderlich has described a peculiar form of asthma, consisting of an attack of gradually increasing dyspnœa, reaching its maximum of intensity in two or three days. At this stage the chest is motionless, fully resonant, and in a state of extreme distention, while the heart is thrust down into the epigastrium, and the liver pushed down in the abdomen.

To me it appears that in these cases the human subject must breathe something after the manner of a reptile; inspiring small gulps of air, and scarcely allowing any expiration, till the lungs become distended with the pent-up air to such an extent that the heart and liver are pushed down in the way described.

Certain it is that the effect of these kinds of attack must be to distend the air-cells of the lung to an unnaturally large size, thus making the human lung like to that of a turtle or other reptile.

Some observers, as Dr. Flint of America, have noticed attacks of asthma associated with elevation of the diaphragm and drawing in of the lower end of the sternum, as if the lung were powerfully contracted and contained but little air; indeed, Dr. Flint says (a), quoting Dr. Walshe, that in some of these cases the volume of the lung may be so much reduced as perceptibly to diminish the clearness of the percussion note. This is the reverse of the state described by Wunderlich, and is a state of lung not often demonstrated, though its possible occurrence is easily understood, and should be borne in mind : it is a condition which, as far as impaired percussion note goes, is not likely to be found where the lungs are emphysematous ; whereas that distension of lung

(a) "On Resp. Organs," p. 364.

from want of contractile power described by Wunderlich will probably be found connected with more or less emphysema, which will be increased the oftener the attacks are repeated.

These variations in the condition of the chest in a fit of asthma serve to explain the differences met with in some of the treatises on medicine, in the descriptions they give of the state of the thorax and abdomen during the fit.

A word may be here said respecting the diagnosis of asthma, a matter of consequence in respect to treatment, and not always so plain as may at first sight appear.

Disease of some parts of the base of the brain will cause attacks of "subjective dyspnœa" that have been mistaken for asthma.

Cases of asthma have been recorded by Gairdner, Heberden, and others, due to organic disease of the brain, and to tumours involving a pressure on the vagus nerve. I have myself observed a case of severe and long-standing dyspnœa due to a tumour pressing on the upper part of the spinal cord.

Dr. Hyde Salter was once called to a distance from town to see an eminent provincial physician ill with attacks resembling asthma, but when examined respiration could be distinctly heard in the chest. This fact, taken with the previous history of the case, pointed to cerebral disorganisation as the true disease, and of this the patient shortly after died.

Attention has been drawn by Fonssagrives and Woillez to attacks of severe paroxysmal dyspnœa, occurring commonly in males from the ages of twenty-four to forty-two, due to engorgement of the bronchial glands. The engorgement may be a simple hypertrophy, or it may arise from tubercular or cancerous disease. The lung symptoms may be thus summed up:—A dry, paroxysmal, suffocating cough ; increasing dyspnœa, accompanied by paroxysms of suffocation,—and during these attacks the respiration is jerking and irregular, and the voice feeble or extinct ; percussion sound clear,—the intra-scapular and upper sternal regions should be carefully examined on this point ; palpation detects increase of the normal thoracic vibrations, and under one or other of the clavicles *frottements*, due to large sonorous râles, audible at some distance, are perceived, and are of much importance. The subacute steady progress of the disease confirms its diagnosis, and its duration varies from fourteen days to six months (*a*).

Tuberculosis of the bronchial glands in children is sometimes a cause of asthmatic fits.

In these cases there is usually a short dry paroxysmal cough, without any whooping or expectoration, there are febrile accessions, with sweating and emaciation; and occasionally examination by percussion of the intra-scapular and supra-sternal regions discloses limited dulness in these parts.

When a child has asthma, and with it most or all of the above symptoms, there is very good reason to think that the paroxysm is due to pressure of an enlarged bronchial gland.

Rarely these cases come to a climax and a

(*a*) Sydenham Society "Year-Book," 1861, p. 193.

cure by the child suddenly expectorating purulent matter ; this continues for a time, then suddenly ceases, the excavated gland cicatrizing and healing.

A small aneurismal tumour within the thorax, pressing on the recurrent nerve, has been known to cause violent spasmodic dyspnœa, with intervals of relief, as in a case of Dr. Barker's in the "St. Thomas's Hospital Reports for 1870."

Certain laryngeal affections—as, for instance, paralysis of the abductors (crico-arytenoidei postici) of the vocal cords, giving rise to dyspnœa and stridulous breathing—must be distinguished from asthma by a laryngoscopic examination, when it will be seen that the vocal cords scarcely separate in inspiration, as they ought to do in a healthy larynx. That complaint of children called Millar's asthma is now well known to be a spasm of the glottis ; the adductor muscles act spasmodically and close the larynx, giving rise to paroxysms of dyspnœa and stridulous breathing.

A few years ago a patient was under my care at the Victoria Park Hospital, who for nine years had been afflicted with what was called asthma, the symptoms resembling those of that complaint. The peculiar sound of her voice, cough, and sneeze made me examine the larynx, and then it was seen that she could not close her larynx in consequence of paralysis of the adductors. Dr. Morell Mackenzie was kind enough to examine this patient, and it was thought there might be an intra-thoracic tumour, but we could not find any sign of one by examination. In his work on nervo-muscular affections of the larynx Dr. Mackenzie has done much to explain the nature of laryngeal dyspnœa.

It will be sufficient to remind the reader that the dyspnœa attendant on heart disease must not be taken for asthma; and though there is a recognised form of asthma due to uterine congestion or irritation, it is scarcely likely that any practitioner, meeting with a case of "cardiac apnœa" in a woman in child-bed, will fail to recognise the danger and gravity of the case before him, and not to imagine he has merely to do with sympathetic asthma.

The prognosis in asthma is generally good, and asthmatics are well known to be generally long-lived; so that invalids who may have been for some time suffering in the chest are wont to feel much satisfaction and comfort when they are assured that their complaint is "only asthma," or is likely to "turn into asthma." The comfort taken by the patient from these assertions is quite legitimate, the truth in these cases being that some lung mischief of a bronchitic, or even of a tuberculous, nature becomes arrested. In the healing process by which the arrest takes place the apex of one lung may become adherent to the chest wall, as is not very rarely observed in arrested consumption; or there may remain thickening of lung tissue or enlargement of bronchi, all causes of attacks of difficulty in the breathing, with accession of cough and expectoration under the influence of atmospheric changes, and yet conditions by no means incompatible with an average duration of life.

Spasmodic asthma, uncomplicated with organic disease, is seldom fatal, but persons have been known now and then to die in the asthmatic fit as from syncope.

Usually when asthma destroys life it is by inducing dilatation of the heart and congestion of the lungs; and as those advanced in years are more prone to these organic changes than young persons, we always look with some anxiety at the case of any elderly person who begins to show signs of asthma. Not long ago I had under observation a gentleman, aged sixty-four, who had become subject to very severe attacks of catarrhal asthma. He had, shortly before I saw him, been assured by more than one of the best authorities in London that he was free from any structural disease, and one physician went so far as to say that the life was one he would not hesitate to recommend for assurance. Gradually, during three subsequent years, the patient's heart became dilated and feeble, and this condition proved ultimately the cause of his death. In young persons who are attacked with asthma the prognosis, though often favourable, must be given only after repeated examinations, and more or less prolonged observation, for asthmatic fits in early life sometimes are the heralds of miliary tubercles in later years. Some months ago I saw a very rapid development of active phthisis take place in a youth who from infancy had been liable to asthmatic attacks.

Feverishness, with increase of temperature and pulse rate, occasional hæmoptysis, and a constantly greater manifestation of physical signs in one lung more than the other during the asthmatic fit, are signs that would lead us to fear the commencement of pulmonary tuberculisation.

CHAPTER III.

Dry and moist asthma—Nature and source of the secretion which takes place.—Hæmoptysis rare ; source of the bleeding when it does occur.—Nervous nature of catarrhal asthma.—A case from Professor Trousseau in illustration.—Nature of hay asthma.—Asthma as contrasted with phthisis. Resemblance between asthma and epilepsy.—Asthma an hereditary disease, alternating often with such diathetic diseases as gout, rheumatism, and some skin affections.—Influence of age in determining prognosis.

ALTHOUGH mention has been made of *dry* as distinct from *moist* asthma, yet it is rare to find an attack of asthma to pass off without some secretion into the air-tubes. When this secretion commences it is a sign that the fit is subsiding, and as the patient begins to cough up small pellets of grey mucus, he gets relief and breathes more freely.

The secretion appears to be an exudation from the bronchial venules, resulting in a measure from the congestion of blood in these vessels caused by the continued muscular spasm to which they have been subjected ; for though a very short attack of asthma may terminate in mucous expectoration, yet when the fit has lasted longer the expectoration is more copious and persistent.

It is rare for hæmorrhage to take place from the lungs in asthma, but it does sometimes occur, and then it is the bronchial venules that furnish the blood which is expectorated.

When the expectoration which commonly terminates a fit of spasmodic asthma is so constant and copious as to become a special point of notice in the case, we have before us an instance of moist or humid asthma, a form of the complaint consequent usually upon a persistence of dry asthma, and often associated with more or less of chronic bronchitis.

In hay asthma, called also summer catarrh, we see an excellent example of catarrhal asthma; so we do also in the asthma due to inhaling ipecacuanha powder, or any other emanation by a susceptible person. The late eminent Professor Trousseau believed catarrhal asthma to be much more common with children than with adults, and quotes a very interesting case of a child who had at times all the symptoms of broncho-pneumonia come on with great suddenness, so that in the short space of one hour abundant subcrepitant rhonchi could be heard all over the chest. The first time Trousseau was called to see this child he treated him energetically with blisters, and in three days the child was well. A few months after a similar attack occurred, and though no active treatment was employed, the child recovered in forty-eight hours. Reflecting upon this rapid recovery, and considering that the mother of this child was very liable to hysteria, Trousseau made up his mind that the attacks were due, not to broncho-pneumonia, but to spasmodic asthma, and the next time he was called to treat his little patient the Professor advised the burning of stramonium leaves in the room; this was done, and the child was perfectly well on the next day. This, therefore, was a good example of a pulmonary neurosis complicated with bronchial secretion, the presence of which

D

had been revealed by the fine subcrepitant mucous rhonchi heard.

Hay asthma is a pulmonary neurosis attended with a profuse flux from the mucous surfaces; and though the complaint may be excited by a cold, yet commonly it so suddenly gains the aeme of its intensity, with sneezing and profuse running from eyes and nose, that it is impossible to view it as other than a true catarrhal neurosis.

I have observed cases of asthma where the catarrh seems to alternate with the dyspnœa; one day the patient wants to know what is to be done for the catarrh, and next time the catarrh is gone,—*cured*, perhaps the patient will say, by something he has been taking, but now the breath is worse than ever. As a sign how little these neurotic attacks are connected with inflammation, there are instances recorded of asthmatics who have actually contracted a sharp attack of bronchitis, and during the course of the complaint have never been troubled at all with their asthma. A striking illustration of this fact has come under my observation while I have been engaged in writing these pages.

The nature of the asthmatic fit, its suddenness of invasion, its prevalence in the heat of summer rather than in the cold of winter, its occasional subsidence, even during an actual attack of real inflammation, confirm us in our view of its essentially nervous nature.

The remarkable histories we have of asthmatic persons fighting for breath in one locality, and perfectly healthy and well almost the very instant they remove to another, further attest the neurotic character of the complaint: the forces and powers are strangely perverted and out of order in asthma, but the tissues themselves are healthy and unchanged. In these respects how powerfully asthma contrasts with pulmonary phthisis! In asthma we see marked and alarming symptoms, and yet there exists no tissue change; in phthisis, with obscure, faintly marked external signs of disease, we may have immense destruction of lung tissue taking place.

In some respects asthma resembles epilepsy, being prone to be excited by any irritation of the system. At times the attacks cease altogether, and it is hoped that the last drug pre-

scribed has cured the complaint, till a sudden
return of the attack under the influence of some
little excitement dissipates the pleasant illusion.
Asthma, too, like some forms of epilepsy, may
be due to the suppression of a skin eruption, or
to gouty or rheumatic poison circulating in the
blood. Like these affections, asthma is un-
questionably an hereditary disease.

In proof of the hereditary and constitutional
nature of asthma, it is not difficult to adduce
instances where children, whose parents have
been liable to gout, have been at a very early
age attacked with asthma; and these cases of
constitutional or diathetic asthma are most
troublesome to deal with. In one case of a boy
aged thirteen years, who had well-marked
attacks of catarrhal asthma, it happened that,
during one period of unusually severe suffering
from cough, expectoration, and difficulty of
breathing, the attack seemed to terminate in a
true purulent expectoration, which, after lasting
a week or two, ceased completely and abruptly,
while careful auscultation gave evident sign of
a small cavity in the situation of the bronchial

glands at the root of the lung. The recovery here was perfect, but the liability to asthma, during the summer more especially, remained as inveterate as before. The parents of this patient had both suffered from gout. Since writing the first edition of this book I have met with a perfectly typical case of spasmodic asthma in a youth, in whose family gout is hereditary.

Trousseau has recorded the case of a Moldavian boy, aged five, who had very distinct fits of asthma, together with some pulmonary emphysema. In his family history there was no mention of gout or rheumatism, and yet two years later this boy had an attack of unmistakable gout in the big toe. During the attack of gout the boy had not a single paroxysm of asthma.

In two cases of well-marked asthma occurring in a brother and sister, and referred to further on (Chap. VI.), the disease was hereditary ; and in the sister the attacks became less frequent and severe when the eruption of psoriasis appeared on her wrists and arms. The brother, too, was liable to an eruption on the skin. I once attended a little girl who had bad eczema of the skin; and when this was cured, well-marked asthmatic attacks came on.

Usually, when asthma comes on in young children of four or five years of age, it is due to an attack of bronchitis or to whooping-cough, and not often to a constitutional diathesis. Examination of the chests of these children will probably reveal signs of emphysema about the apices of the lungs caused by the violent paroxysms of cough driving the air into the upper part of the lungs when it cannot escape, owing to closure of the glottis.

Under these circumstances of local origin we may look to the child growing out of the disease.

It is curious to observe how early in life true asthma may make its appearance. Dr. Salter observed eleven cases in the first year of existence, and sixty during the first ten years of life. From ten to twenty years the number of cases occurring was thirty; and from thirty to forty years, forty-four; the numbers then diminishing rapidly during the following decades of existence. In examining an asthmatic infant care should be taken to see that the dyspnœa is bronchial and not laryngeal; and an opportunity should be obtained of examining the small patient when free from actual dyspnœa, to see if there be any sign of tuberculisation of the bronchial glands, or of emphysema of the lung. That this last complaint may become fully developed generally, in a child of one or two years old I have often observed; but there may be well-marked emphysema without much spasm, the symptoms being rather those of chronic bronchitis, and we are told the child has had a cough and cold from its birth. Emphysema and asthma are both diseases of proved hereditary nature, but either may exist independently of the other.

When asthma develops thus early in life and independently of any whooping-cough or bronchitis, we may assume that the constitutional or diathetic tendency to the disease is strong, and all the resources of medicine, climate and regimen must be set in force, and then we may hope to see the child outgrow the tendency to the disease. Sometimes the constitutional proclivity to asthma does not manifest itself till the age of eighteen or twenty, and then on going into some new locality, the individual is suddenly attacked with a fit of asthma, and wonders what is the matter with him; he suspects he has taken a cold till additional experience causes the real truth to dawn upon him.

A patient, sent to me by Dr. Kavanagh, of New Cross, had asthma attack him suddenly just in the way above described, at the age of sixteen, when he chanced to be at Freshwater, in the Isle of Wight. This gentleman, when a child, had a troublesome eruption on the skin, which, after some time, disappeared, apparently to make way for the asthma.

In these cases where diathetic but uncomplicated asthma develops thus later in life, the prognosis is less favourable than when it comes on in babyhood, as the tendency to tissue change increases with age.

In those advanced in life asthmatic attacks are commonly due to some organic change in the lungs or heart, and though much relief may be afforded by treatment, yet a permanent cure is very doubtful.

CHAPTER IV.

Treatment of dry and catarrhal asthma.—Position, atmosphere, and other simple measures to be used to prevent the invasion of the fit.—If these fail, other means to be at once employed.—Inhalations of burning nitre paper, of chloroform and nitrite of amyl ; use of the inhaling pipe of Mr. Bird.—Various kinds of medicated papers and cigarettes.—Use of internal remedies during the fit of asthma.—Tinctures of Datura tatula, of stramonium, belladonna, sumbul, cannabis.—Use of chloral, &c.—Perles of ether.—Hypodermic injections.

ENOUGH has now been said as to the nature and causes of spasmodic asthma to show on what principles our treatment must be based— be it for purposes of prevention, alleviation, or cure. We must not lose sight of the essentially nervous character of asthma, even in its catarrhal form, and our treatment must be rather that for a spasmodic neurosis than for an inflammatory catarrh.

There are certain sensations, the meaning of which the tried asthmatic soon learns by painful

experience rightly to interpret, which show that
a fit of asthma is coming on. Thus, the individual may be irritable and restless, or perhaps
heavy for sleep ; often there is itching of some
part of the body, as, for instance, of the nose
or eyes, and a peculiar itching under the chin
is a marked premonition of the asthmatic
seizure. In some persons flatulence and dyspepsia usher in the fit, though they may have
been discreet in their diet.

The best methods for averting a threatening
attack of asthma are very much matters of
individual experience, but yet there are certain
general principles which to some extent guide
us in dealing with all cases. We should try
to promote the respiratory action by placing
the patient with his elbows and arms resting on
some fixed point, so that the muscles of the
arms and shoulders may help to expand the
chest. Sometimes emotional excitement, or
some strong effort on the part of the patient,
whereby the attention is diverted, will avert
the paroxysm. Dr. Salter tells us of one case
where a lady could stave off her asthmatic fit

by sitting down at once to the piano, and of another instance of one who had his asthma stopped at once by being put on a horse which ran away with him. Seeing how profoundly asthma is influenced by atmospheric conditions, it is well for the asthmatic, provided he be yet able to move, to try getting from one room to another on a different level, or to go out of doors. If he suffer specially in a dry air, then let the air of his room be made moist by having a kettle placed on the fire, and allowing the steam to escape into the air of the chamber.

Hearing of the good that many cases of asthma appear to derive from breathing compressed air, one would suggest a compressed air chamber as a valuable addition to the premises of the asthmatic patient. M. Bertin, who has had some experience of this way of treating asthma, states that, out of ninety-two cases of old standing asthma, sixty-seven were quite cured by means of the inhalation of compressed air. These would probably be cases of asthma complicated with emphysema of the lungs, and the "modus operandi" of com-

pressed air in these cases will be alluded to
further on.

It is known that in some cases of emphysema among men working in diving-bells, the
man has felt ease and comfort while down in
the bell breathing a very condensed atmosphere. The way in which a permanent cure of
old emphysema is to be brought about by this
means is not very easy of comprehension,
though the fact that temporary relief is obtained in many cases cannot be doubted.

A loaded state of the stomach or bowels
must be properly attended to and relieved by
an emetic or purgative ; and if the feet be cold,
they should be at once placed in hot mustard
and water.

To one liable to gout and acidity, a draught
should be given containing a scruple of bicar-
bonate of soda or potash, with half a drachm
of aromatic spirit of ammonia, in a wineglassful
of peppermint water. In another case, a
tumbler half full of *very hot* brandy, gin, or
whisky, with water, may be found effective in
giving relief. Hot coffee, also, without milk,
is a well-known and very efficacious remedy.

If, despite the employment of these simple means to avert the paroxysm, it nevertheless increases, the patient's words become fewer and shorter, his face congested, and his chest difficulty very great, he should at once resort to the inhalation of the fumes of burning nitre paper; or, if this be not at hand, he need not hesitate to try a few whiffs of chloroform.

The speedy and decided relief obtained from the inhalation of chloroform in a fit of spasmodic asthma has now been long recognised. In the *Medical Times* for December, 1847, is published an interesting case, by Mr. Chandler, of a lady, aged 56, who for twenty years had been subject to attacks of spasmodic asthma, for the relief of which "the resources of the 'Pharmacopœia' had been exhausted in vain." On December 6th, after an attack of the then prevalent influenza, this lady was seized with her asthma, with extreme dyspnœa, great sense of constriction, and acute darting pains through the chest and epigastrium.

Half a drachm of chloroform was now administered on a sponge; after a while unconsciousness came on, with relaxation of the limbs, and, as she lay back in the bed, the inspirations became prolonged and deep, with considerable intervals.

There was no return of the spasm, and the patient remained comparatively well, feeling no ill effect from the inhalation. The vapour of sulphuric ether had been previously tried in this case, but it seemed to increase the sufferings of the patient.

Employed with due caution at the onset of an asthmatic fit, a very small quantity of chloroform vapour will often suffice to avert the coming mischief; and, where the asthma is purely spasmodic, there seems reason to believe that this practice of checking the onset of the fit by a little chloroform may in time break through the habit entirely.

When the chloroform is entrusted to the individual patient, my practice is to recommend the use of one of Bird's inhaling pipes (*a*) as a

(*a*) A full description, with illustration, of this useful inhaling pipe, invented by Mr. Bird, of Seymour Street, W., will be found in the *British Medical Journal*, vol. i., 1869, as well as in the *Medical Times and Gazette* of same date. The pipe is made by Maw, of Aldersgate Street.

safeguard against accidents. Ten drops of chloroform, with half a drachm of spirit of wine or of camphor, should be poured on the felt sponge, and this inserted into the bowl of the pipe, so that the vapour may be inhaled through the tube. Should the vapour overpower the patient's consciousness, he will be almost sure to let the pipe fall from his hand; but, with the small dose of chloroform above indicated, it is not very likely that consciousness will be lost.

In a few rare instances chloroform fails to relieve, if it does not actually increase, the distress of the patient; and, after frequent repetitions of a large dose, the system may become less susceptible to its influence, so that the dose has to be increased till patients find themselves consuming this anæsthetic in a way that is astounding. It is always important to begin, therefore, with a very small dose of from five to ten drops on a handkerchief, or in the inhaling pipe, and not to increase the dose without good cause for so doing.

Recently the amber-coloured liquid, smelling like the essence of ripe pears, and known as Nitrite of Amyl, has been used with great benefit as a speedy means of obtaining relief in spasmodic asthma, as well as in some forms of cardiac neurosis and spasm.

Nitrite of amyl has been shown by Dr. Richardson to act by causing paralysis of the organic nerves, which govern the contractility of the blood vessels; it is, therefore, a relaxer of muscular and arterial spasm.

When five drops of Nitrite of Amyl are inhaled, there is increase of pulse rate, throbbing of carotids, and flushing of the face, with feeling of tension. These effects follow in about thirty or forty seconds, the action of the inhalation rapidly causing dilatation of the blood vessels.

The nitrite has been given subcutaneously, and by the mouth; but the best way to use it in asthma is to drop five drops on a piece of lint, and hold it before the nostrils of the patient for a few seconds, till the pulse begins to increase and the face to flush (*a*). This remedy

---

(*a*) Dr. Talfourd Jones, in the *Practitioner* for October, 1871, has recorded excellent results from the use of the Nitrite of Amyl in asthma.

should only be had in small quantities at a time, as it soon completely loses its power by keeping.

Of the value of inhalations of the smoke from the Datura Stramonium and Datura Tatula it is hardly necessary to say much, so well are these remedies known, both to the Profession and the public. The old-fashioned way of smoking the chopped-up stramonium in a pipe with tobacco is now in a great measure superseded by the cigarettes which are made with camphor and stramonium; and of these, those that are prepared from the leaves of the Datura Tatula, first introduced into use by Messrs. Savory and Moore are, in my experience, both safe and effective. Several asthmatic patients under my own care feel that the use of one of these cigarettes whenever they feel the fit impending, averts, or greatly mitigates their distress, and adds much to the comfort of their lives.

In using the fumes of stramonium for the relief of hay asthma, it is a good plan to take the inhalation in a concentrated form, after the plan recommended by Mr. Lawford. The

E

herb is to be washed and dried, and then smoked, the smoke being puffed into an inverted ale-glass; when this is full it is to be placed over the mouth, and a deep inspiration taken. The result is a momentary sense of suffocation, then copious expectoration of ropy mucus and immediate relief.

The cigars made with the rolled-up leaves of the stramonium are not more efficacious, and hardly so safe to use as the camphorated cigarettes; but, whatever form the patient may use, it is well at once to stop the inhalation of the smoke as soon as any feeling of faintness and giddiness comes on; inattention on this point has led to serious and even fatal consequences from smoking stramonium leaves in an ordinary pipe.

In the well-known Espic Cigarette, solanaceous and other plants are combined together, according to the following formula :—

R   Folii Belladonnæ, gr. vj.;
  ,,   Hyoscyami, gr. iij.;
  ,,   Stramonii, gr. iij.;
  ,,   Phellandrii aquatici, gr. j.;
    Extracti opii, gr. ⅓.;
    Aquæ lauro cerasi, qs.
The powdered leaves are wetted with the ext. opii. dissolved in the laurel water, then dried, and put up in cigarettes.

I have met with patients who get prompt relief from these cigarettes, and from these alone, others having little or no effect in relieving them.

The cigarettes, made by Mr. Slade, of Long Acre, I have tried in cases of troublesome asthma, and find patients to speak well of them.

Useful cigarettes are made of the nitre paper already mentioned in the following way.

White blotting-paper is cut into small slips about seven inches long, and one and a half broad; these are soaked in a solution, made by dissolving four ounces of nitre in half a pint of hot water, then dried and rolled round a pencil to give them a cigarette form, and are at once ready for use.

The nitre paper, made with a saturated solution, can also be kept in squares ready for burning in the patient's room, or in the inhaling pipe; and when the room is well filled with the fumes of the burning paper, the asthmatic is almost sure of obtaining relief. In one case under my observation, nitre paper burnt in the patient's bed room will prevent the asthmatic attack without awakening him; if one is at hand who can ignite the paper as soon as ever difficult respiration in the sleeper shows that his enemy is near at hand. In some cases of very obstinate asthma, the addition of one quarter of a grain of arsenious acid in solution to each of the nitre cigarettes is an immense advantage; a few full and deep inhalations from such a cigarette once or twice in the day tend to promote the permanent cure of many forms of asthma.

There are various other ways of medicating the nitre paper; as, for instance, by washing it over with the compound tincture of benzoin, or by adding to the solution some of the solution of nitrate of mercury, in such proportion as to have two grains of the nitrate in each cigarette. These balsamic and mercurial cigarettes are, however, of more marked service in some chronic affections of the throat and larynx than in asthma. For the prevention and alleviation of hay asthma, the use of tobacco in cigars or in a pipe is a remedy of known and proved value. Nitre paper is, I believe, the basis of the "Papier Fruneau" so valuable in asthma, and also of a very useful paper prepared by Mr. Dowling, of Exeter, which I have often used with excellent results.

Although ammonia is not a sedative, yet at times the fumes of ammonia inhaled may break the asthmatic paroxysm. The practice of applying solution of ammonia, mixed with an equal quantity of water, on a brush to the posterior part of the pharynx, was introduced some years ago by Duclos, and he claimed to have effected wonderful cures by this practice. It is a method of treatment to be tried with the utmost caution, for the first touch of the saturated brush on the wall of the pharynx will at times cause a paroxysm of suffocation that is dangerous and alarming, though afterwards the patient may remain for a time free from asthmatic fits.

In using any kind of inhalation, whether by pipe, cigarette, or inhaling jug, it is necessary to understand that the medicated vapour should be fairly drawn into the lungs, and not merely puffed in and out of the mouth after the method of those who smoke tobacco.

A want of attention to this point often causes patients to complain of the failure of medicated cigarettes to give them any relief, but when they once acquire the habit of fairly inhaling the vapour, they soon see reason to alter their opinion. In those very excellent French cigarettes known as the Cigarettes de Joy, sold by Wilcox, of Oxford Street, brief but very plain directions are given to teach the patient how to use them, and, when properly used, they are remarkably efficacious in relieving asthma in all its forms.

I have already made mention of some of the more ordinary internal remedies to be had recourse to with a view to stopping an impending fit of asthma; such, for instance, as strong coffee, hot spirits and water, alkaline draughts, and so forth. I now come to say a few words on such medicines as may be employed during the actual fit for the sake of relieving the patient. Anti-spasmodics are the only medicines that appear to me worth swallowing for

any relief that may be obtained, and of these
I always use first the tincture of the Datura
Tatula. When called to a patient in a state
of severe dyspnœa, with wheezy noises audible
all over the chest, and quite unable to lie
down, or indeed to remain long easy in any
one position, my plan is at once to advise a
stramonium cigarette, or some nitre paper
rolled up and burnt in Bird's inhaling pipe.
Then, as an internal remedy, the following is
one that I have proved to be deserving of
confidence :—

> R Tinct. Daturæ Tatulæ, ℼ x.—xx.;
> Sodæ bicarb., gr. x.—xx.;
> Spir. chlorof., ℼ xv., vel. spir. ætheris, ℼ xxx.;
> Aq. camphoræ, f. ℥j. M. Ft. Hst.

This draught may be taken every one, two,
three, or four hours, according to the urgency
of the symptoms.

Tincture of Stramonium may be substituted
for the tincture of the Tatula, but is not so
efficacious, being more narcotic and less anti-
spasmodic than the Datura Tatula. Belladonna
I find valuable as a useful anti-spasmodic in

asthma, especially given at night in a full dose. Like stramonium, belladonna appears to quicken the respiration, sometimes belladonna appears to surpass stramonium as a reliever of the spasmodic form of asthma.

In very troublesome dyspnœa, due to old-standing cardiac disease, with lividity of face and congested surface generally, I have found the tincture of belladonna, in doses of seven drops three times a day, give an amount of relief, and reduce the congested look of the face and surface in a very decided and satis-factory way, surpassing entirely the very numerous list of remedies that had been tried previously.

I recommend belladonna in cases of dys-pnœa with much congestion, where opium is little else than a veritable poison to the patient.

The dose should be small at first, say five drops of the tincture, but if this does not seem to affect the patient soon, the dose should be quickly increased, and it is often not till we are giving six to ten drops in the dose that we get curative effects. If the belladonna be given in pill, a very good combination is made, thus—

> ℞ Ext. belladonnæ, gr. ⅓.;
> Pulv. radicis belladonnæ, gr. ⅓. Mix.

This pill may be given at bedtime.

The tincture of the seeds of stramonium of the " Ph. Brit." is a good and efficient medicine, and may be given in doses of ten to twenty drops. The extract of the seeds is five times stronger than the extract made from the leaves, and the spirituous extract of "Ph. Brit." is a more stable preparation than the water extract of the " Ph. Lond.," and may be given in a pill containing from a quarter of a grain upwards.

If the asthmatic be complaining much of flatus in the bowels, then if he can be persuaded to swallow a small teaspoonful of the sp. ammoniæ fœtidus in a wineglass of mint water, or brandy and water, it will probably be for his relief and comfort.

Among other remedies may be named the tinctures of cannabis, of sumbul, and of henbane. They are rarely preferable to the stramonium for medicinal efficacy, but at times one may be glad to use one or other for a change. The tincture of sumbul, in doses of fifteen to twenty drops, is an elegant, pleasant medicine, and certainly possesses decided antispasmodic properties; like the other tinctures, it will go well in a mixture with ether or spiritus chloroformi. The Hydrate of Chloral in doses of fifteen grains and more sometimes relieves asthma in a wonderful way, but like many other remedies it cannot always be depended on.

The croton chloral hydrate, so valuable in my experience in neuralgia of the fifth nerve, does not disturb the brain so much as the ordinary chloral, and might well be tried in asthma. At present I have not any experience, however, of its use to offer to the reader.

Among very convenient internal medicines I may here mention Clertan's "perles," made by M. Jozeau, of the Haymarket, and those made also by M. Tisy, of Paris, and kept in London by Messrs. Corbyn.

These perles are thin gelatine capsules containing a few drops of ether, chloroform, phosphorated oil, or any other liquid medicine. They can be carried about easily, and one or two of the ether perles swallowed will often quickly relieve an attack of commencing spasm and dyspnœa.

Before quitting the subject of the immediate treatment of the paroxysm of asthma, a word may be said on the use of subcutaneous injections as a means of affording relief. The effect of the subcutaneous injection of morphia was tried some years ago, with marked success, by Hirtz, in the case of a girl who had severe attacks of asthma, the respiration being so noisy as to be audible outside the room.

One hundredth of a gramme of acetate of morphia injected under the skin of the arm gave the greatest relief in five minutes.

For rapidity, but not for safety of action, however, the sulphate of atropine, in doses of one five-hundredth of a gramme, was found superior to the morphia.

It is suggested, in chronic cases, to try the two remedies in alternation. (*Bull. Gén. de Thérap.*)

For precautions requisite in making and using solutions of morphia, atropia, and strychnia for subcutaneous purposes, I would refer the reader to Dr. Anstie's remarks in the *Practitioner* for July, 1868.

I would venture to hope that some useful hints may be gathered from this chapter as to the means to be employed for the relief of the asthmatic when in the actual fit. The next chapter is on the management of the asthmatic, with a view to a permanent cure.

CHAPTER V.

Management of the asthmatic patient in the intervals of his attacks, with a view to a curative effect.—Certain nerve-tonic medicines of use.—Caprice of asthma with respect to atmospheric causes prevents our laying down any absolute directions as to climate.—As a rule, the air of towns, most generally agreeable, cause of this.—Of exercise and diet.—Medicinal treatment.—Tonics often of great service.—Cases illustrating effects of treatment.

WHEN a patient has recovered from the distress of a bad fit of asthma, he naturally inquires, "What can I do to prevent these dreadful attacks?" In answer, we may assure him that he can do a very great deal to avert the fits if he will but exercise some resolution, and not rest content that he is doing all that can be done in swallowing two tablespoonfuls of physic three times a day, and taking pills every night.

That certain medicines of the nerve-tonic class—such as zinc, quinine, arsenic, phos-

phorus, and salts of iron and silver—do act
very powerfully and unmistakeably as remedies
for asthma, I have repeatedly proved in a
goodly number of cases; but, such is the noto-
rious caprice of asthma, that we often fail, even
after trying remedies that experience leads us
to think promise well, thoroughly to cure the
complaint by our medicines; and, hence, it is
that it becomes of such great importance to
point out to the patient certain rules of living,
which he must carry out faithfully if he really
wish to keep free from his troublesome complaint.

With respect, first of all, to the climate
adapted for the residence of a person liable to
spasmodic asthma. This is so entirely and
peculiarly a matter of individual experience,
that it is vain to attempt to lay down any
universal and absolute law upon the subject.
General experience would, I expect, make out
the city of London to be the spot most agreeable to the majority of asthmatics.

I believe it is the carbonaceous matter or
the London air that renders it so salutary and

anti-spasmodic; for the more sooty the air, the better does the asthmatic seem to be. In a case to be mentioned shortly, carbon given internally was of use, though of course it could not come into actual contact with the air-vesicles of the lung. (Case X., chapter vi.)

As a rule, dust is specially obnoxious to asthmatic persons; some kinds being far worse than others. Thus, the dust of hay or of corn is a powerful exciter of asthma; so, too, is the dust of linseed meal or of ipecacuanha, the pollen of certain flowers, and, in a less degree, the dust from carpets and house furniture.

With respect to temperature, a sudden fall is a potent cause of asthma; so, when cold sets in suddenly, the asthmatic must protect his chest and respiratory organs by a comforter, or silk handkerchief, and this last forms an excellent respirator.

Sea air is peculiarly bad for some, while others, especially those subject to hay asthma, or summer catarrh, are much relieved by it; moisture in the air, soothing to some, is very oppressive to others. The rooms inhabited by the asthmatic should be lofty and airy, and when warmed this should be done by an open fire, and never by a stove or by hot-water pipes. Candles are better than gas as a means of lighting the apartment. The bedroom must be kept well aired, and the asthmatic must take care that his mattress and pillow are not stuffed with anything that may prove a cause of his fit assailing him as soon as his bed gets warm. Sometimes a feather bed will prove an efficient maintainer of a tendency to nocturnal asthma. Daily exercise in the open air should not be neglected; and several cases testify to the effect of a steady walk in preventing an attack of asthma even when it already threatens. Horse exercise is especially beneficial, it promotes regular movement of the diaphragm, and it is, in my opinion, the best form of exercise the asthmatic can indulge in.

The dietetic management of asthma is a point on which universal experience teaches that much stress should be laid ; and here it is that the patient must exercise some amount of resolution and self-denial.

In the first place, he must avoid any special articles of food that prove indigestible and provocative of asthma to his individual constitution, and he must further avoid anxiously anything like excess of food and over-loading of the stomach. A distended stomach acts mechanically by its pressure upwards against that very important respiratory muscle the diaphragm, to embarrass the free action of the heart and lungs, besides being also a source of reflex irritation to the system generally. If, however, the overloaded stomach does not happen thus to become an immediate exciter of the asthmatic fit, the probability is that the acidity and flatulence likely to be generated in the imperfect digestion of a large mass of aliment will most certainly bring on before long an attack of asthma likely to prove severe and persistent.

The digestive powers of asthmatic patients are, as a rule, weak ; hence they must never be over-taxed, and it is a point of some moment to see that the asthmatic is not allowed to take much food when under the immediate influence, of any excess of fatigue. He must rest quietly

F

and then begin to take food slowly and sparingly, using for drink either weak brandy and water or else dry Manzanilla sherry. In the general mode of living, it is the best for asthmatic persons to make their chief meal in the middle of the day, from one to three o'clock, and to try and take little or nothing after this unless it be some bread and milk, or a cup of cocoa or tea with plenty of milk in it, not later than six o'clock.

The dinner should consist of some wholesome meat, as mutton, beef, or fowl; boiled fish, too, may be allowed, and so may a light pudding. Cheese, pie, and pudding-crusts are notoriously bad, and must be carefully avoided, as should also dessert.

But little drink should be taken with dinner; but two or three hours after the meal some toast and water or pale brandy and water may be allowed.

Malt liquors of all kinds are bad, and should be avoided.

Dining thus early in the day ensures the completion of the digestive process before the patient goes to bed, and very greatly diminishes the severity of nocturnal asthma, if it does not entirely prevent the attack coming on.

In the morning, it is to be hoped the patient will have a fair appetite, and breakfast is the meal when this may be indulged with least risk of mischief. Coffee or tea, with eggs, mutton chops, cold meat, or game, are allowable on the breakfast-table of the asthmatic.

By this practice of taking a good breakfast and an early dinner of wholesome food, with little or nothing during the after part of the day, it is surprising with what comfort an asthmatic can get through his nights. To submit to this strict regimen always requires some determination, and many persons, especially those who have free expectoration with their asthma, have the very erroneous belief that anything short of three good meals of meat in a day is a dietary quite insufficient to enable them to bear up against the presumed weakness and exhaustion which must, as they suppose, accrue on protracted attacks of asthma and expectoration. I never yet knew or heard of one patient of this

class who was not made in every respect worse
by this bad practice of high feeding, with the
liberal alcoholic stimulation which is sure to go
along with it. The reason of this is, that owing
to the high feeding much blood is made, and
this stagnates and congests in the pulmonary
capillaries which can only relieve themselves by
secretion of mucus, and thus copious expectoration is kept up by the constant high
feeding.

To see what good results can be obtained by
a severely strict plan of diet and regimen, any
one need only peruse the cases published by
Mr. Pridham, of Bideford. One case, first pub-,
lished in the *British Medical Journal* for 1860
is a most impressive one. A clergyman, 70
years of age, had been asthmatic for ten years.
He was not able to lie down in bed, and for
years every night he had anticipated death
before morning; when, however, a copious,
heavy expectoration had been thrown off the
lungs, he was relieved, and was able to get up
and move about in much discomfort.

His diet was as follows :—At six in the morning, a cup of coffee ; at nine, he had tea or coffee, toast, eggs, or a chop ; lunch at one, on bread, cheese, and porter ; afterwards a good substantial dinner, followed by both tea and supper !

This patient, despite his rather forcible remonstrances, was persuaded to take off three-quarters of the total amount of food taken in the twenty-four hours. The result was, that at the end of a week he could lie down and sleep ; and, while his expectoration decreased, his appetite improved nicely. This improvement continued, and in due time he became able to lie down and sleep during the whole night, as well as to resume the clerical duties which had been for ten years suspended.

This is a well-marked and interesting case for the encouragement of the asthmatic to persevere in habits of self-denial and care in eating and drinking.

In the *Medical Times and Gazette* for Feb. 1870, is an account of the Abbot of La Trappe, who was a bad asthmatic till he was submitted to the extremely rigid diet of the convent, involving abstinence from meat, and then he quite lost his asthma.

The system of diet which Mr. Pridham recommends for a confirmed asthmatic is as follows : it is certainly a rigid one, but of its curative properties, in many inveterate cases of asthma, there seems good evidence.

> *Breakfast, at eight a.m.*, to consist of half a pint of tea or coffee, with cream, and two ounces of stale bread.
>
> *Dinner at one.*—Two ounces of beef or mutton, and two ounces of dry stale bread or boiled rice. Three hours after dinner, half a pint of brandy and water (weak), or sherry and water; or else toast and water *ad libitum*.
>
> *Supper at seven.*—Two ounces of meat and two ounces of bread.

As a general rule, I prefer to allow the patient a moderate dinner at two or three o'clock, and then to dispense with supper entirely, though a small quantity of toast, or bread with butter may be taken at tea-time.

Many patients will be content, and do very

comfortably on this restricted system of diet, but others are met with, true asthmatics, to whom rather more licence must be given, or they will get into a weak and highly nervous state very adverse to throwing off the asthmatic tendency.

To these cases we must allow a larger number of meals, taking care that they never at any one time have more than from six to eight ounces of food, and as a rule the food should be of a fleshy or nitrogenous character rather than farinaceous or saccharine.

In some of these cases, where debility is an obvious symptom, I do not hesitate to advise a cup of milk, with brandy, during the night, as a means of preventing great exhaustion.

Beef tea, with pepsine powder or pepsine wine, is also a capital food in the daytime in these cases.

When the patient, however, recovers his strength, and the volume of blood circulating in the body and the lungs increases, then it will be requisite to cut down the diet a little, or there will certainly be premonitions of the return of the attacks of breath-difficulty. The quantity and quality of the blood, as well as of the air going through the lungs of the asthmatic, require to be adjusted to a nicety; disturbance in the balance of these two circulations is sure to cause difficult breathing.

When we have managed the important, but often difficult matter of getting the asthmatic patient to abide by a regular system of diet, and when a short experience has proved to the patient that he is *not being lowered*, but, on the other hand, *manifestly invigorated*, both in body and mind, by what may at first appear to one who has been a high feeder rather scanty fare, then is the time to endeavour by medicines to overcome the asthmatic tendency in the constitution.

The medicines that appear to me most generally useful in overcoming the tendency to asthma are of the tonic and nervine class; thus, iron, quinine, mineral acids, silver, zinc, arsenic, with many others, possess good claim to our notice.

To give a tonic during the day, and an anti-spasmodic at night, I often find a successful practice, as the following case shows :—

CASE I.—Sarah H——, æt. 22, living at Limehouse, came to the Victoria Park Hospital, in the summer, in consequence of attacks of asthma. Her mother died of this disease, and she has two brothers, between 20 and 30, who are great sufferers, and in whom the asthmatic physique is already developed, though this is not the case with the patient, who is well made, and of healthy, rather florid aspect.

She has been ill two years, and is worst in damp weather, always has some amount of dyspnœa, but the worst attacks come on when in bed.

There is no history of gout or rheumatism in the family, nor of any skin disease.

Chest, fully resonant ; breathing, feeble. No râle or rhonchus. Tongue, moist. Pulse, 74. Bowels, not open.

This patient for the space of five weeks took no other medicine than a grain of Extr. stramonii every night, and a mixture of—

Ferri Sulph., gr. j.
Mag. Sulph., ℈j.
Aq. Menth. Pip., ʒj.

three times daily. At the end of this time she declared herself to be free from difficulty in the breathing, and was discharged cured.

The tendency in this case clearly is to an emphysematous state of lung; the constant sense of dyspnœa and hereditary nature of the disease pointed to this ; and it is in these cases where iron preparations are so very beneficial.

Asthma due to bronchitis ; spasm a feature in the case, long course of treatment, and at last complete cure by oxide of silver.

CASE. II.—Isaac P., æt. 24, a pale dark youth, has been some time under treatment for cough and difficult breathing, the result of a severe cold caught six months ago.

Seen by me August 5th, 1867. He has just come back from Hastings, and while there had very little cough and very little asthma, but since his return to the vicinity of London his cough has returned, and at night he has sudden and bad attacks of difficulty in the breathing.

The chest resonance is good, breathing feeble, skin cool, pulse quiet.

℞ Ext. Stramonii, gr. j. om. nocte.
and mixture of phosphoric acid, ether, and mint water,
three times daily.

August 12th.—Much relieved ; rests well.

August 19th.—Worse, breath very bad ; add to mixture, tr. lobel. ether, ℳ xv.

I did not see him again until September 23rd, when he came to me quite as bad as he was when first seen ; he says the stramonium pill has lost all its effect; and at night he starts up with sudden attacks of dyspnœa, pallor of face, abdomen strongly drawn in at epigastrium. The pulse is weak, but no cardiac disease to be detected.

From October 7th till 21st he took, twice daily, a pill containing gr. ¼th of oxide of silver, and a mixture with some dilute nitric acid, and this treatment told at once on his asthma, so that at the end of October he seemed to be perfectly cured.

This was a complex case. The origin of the asthma was bronchitis ; the mild air of Hastings gave immense relief, but it was a nervine tonic medicine that did, in this case, act quite as a specific ; and I ought to say that I never before saw such marked effect produced by oxide of silver, though I have given it in numerous cases with a certain amount of benefit.

Spasmodic asthma after bronchitis, relieved by oxide of silver, cured by arsenic.

CASE III.—Charles W., æt. 36, has been liable to asthma for two years since he got wet. The attacks come on very early in the morning, and pass off with cough and expectoration of clear mucus. Chest resonant, heart sounds feeble generally.

> ℞ Argenti Oxidi, gr. j.;
> Ext. Lupuli, gr. ij.

This pill was taken at bed-time with speedy

relief. One night he omitted the pill, and the attack at 3 a.m. was as bad as ever.

He kept well for some time, but, after taking cold, the asthma returned, and the pills failed to relieve; a change was therefore made to the liquor arsenicalis, three drops three times a day in infus. calumbæ. Under this medicine he got quite well.

Arsenious acid and the liquor arsenicalis (Fowler's Solution), which is arsenious acid dissolved by carbonate of potash, are both valuable remedies in the cure of spasmodic asthma.

The arsenious acid may be given in a granule or pill made with manna, in a dose of 1-50th to 1-20th of a grain with perfect safety, and the liquor arsenicalis may be given in a dose of ♏ ij. to ♏ viij., the larger dose representing gr. 1-16th of arsenious acid.

The liquor sodæ arseniatis, which contains a definite arseniate of soda in the proportion of four grains to the ounce, is also a good preparation, and may agree better with the stomach than the arsenious acid preparations.

The following cases illustrate the effect of arsenic as a remedy for asthma:—

Spasmodic asthma of ten years' standing.— Great relief from Fowler's solution.

CASE IV.—*October 25th*, 1866.—Edward G—, æt. 33, came to the hospital. Been liable to asthma for ten years ; from age of twelve had a cough and shortness of breath. At times is free for some weeks of all breath difficulty. Face cheerful, pale, no congested look. Heart and lungs good. Not worse in damp weather ; always breathes best when in London ; lives at Bethnal Green.

The attacks come on about four a.m., with sense of tightness across chest, and go off with cough and mucous expectoration.

Never any hæmoptysis, gout, rheumatism, or skin disease.

R Hst. Ferri et quassiæ c. mag. sulph., Əj. t. d. s.
Pil. conii co., o. n. s.

November 1st.—"In statu quo" in all respects Pt. omnia.

November 8th.—Worse. Had a bad attack.

R Liq. Fowleri, ℥iij., ex inf. calumbæ, t. d s.
Pt. Pil.

Once or twice feared an attack was coming for the first week, but persevered with the medicine, and on November 29th felt well enough to be discharged, greatly relieved. In this case, the intervals of perfect freedom from breath difficulties should be noticed as a favourable element in the case.

In the uncomplicated asthma of children the

Fowler's Solution is often very serviceable. I select one from among many instances in proof:

Spasmodic asthma in a boy cured by liquor arsenicalis.

CASE V.—Henry W., æt. 10 years, a fair lad, was sent to me at Victoria Park Hospital by Dr. Borlase Hicks.

The boy has bad attacks of nocturnal asthma, obliging him to sit up at night; he is worse in hot weather, but gets relief when at the sea-side. He has a good deal of cough; wheezy sounds with very prolonged expiration are audible over his chest. Tongue clean and moist.

He once had eczema of the scalp, and as this eruption got well the asthma developed itself.

Belladonna and bromide of ammonium gave no relief whatever, but during the month of July when his attacks were at the worst, I put him on small doses of the liquor arsenicalis with speedy and most decided relief to all his bad symptoms.

The presence of some amount of bronchitis and gastric disturbance need not prevent the curative action of the arsenical solution.

Severe attacks of asthma of long standing, with chronic bronchitis. Complete cure by Fowler's solution.

CASE VI.—In the following case, the curative

effect of Fowler's solution was both prompt and permanent.

On July 7th, 1864, at the end of a rather heavy afternoon's work at the hospital, a patient, looking the picture of misery from chronic chest troubles, came to me for advice.

Her age was about 50, and her complaint was of cough and much yellow expectoration, with extreme dyspnœa, debility, loss of appetite, and frequent vomiting of her meals.

The chest was tender but resonant, respiration very feeble. Tongue red edged and furred in centre. This patient was ready with a long account of the advice she had had and the amount of physic she had taken, but, not having time left to hear all this, I advised her to take the following draught three times daily, with the pill at night, and come to me again in a week :

R Hst. Calumbæ c Soda
Liq. Fowleri, ᵐij., t. d. s.
Pil conii co., gr. v. om. nocte.

In a week's time the relief to all the symptoms was most remarkable ; she continued the treatment till the hospital letter was out, and on May 27th, 1867, I saw her looking stout and healthy ; and she said she had not needed any treatment since she left Victoria Park Hospital, in August, 1864.

Complicated asthma.—Symptoms aggravated by arsenical solution.—Relief by other remedies.

CASE VII.—Mrs. Mary B——, æt. about 50,

has been attending at Victoria Park Hospital
for ten years, in consequence of great difficulty
in the breathing, with dark expectoration, at
times mixed with blood.

Stout, not unhealthy in aspect, has severe cardiac palpitation at night. No murmur heard.
Ordered, on February 20th, 1866, to take—

> Liquor Fowleri, ♏ij., ter die.

March 1st.—Much worse. The spitting of
blood has been very troublesome. Omit the
medicine, and take the following :—

> Sodæ hypophos., gr. v.
> Sodæ bicarb., 'gr. v.
> Aq. menth. pip., ʒj., m. t. d. s.
> Pil. Zinci et hyoscyami, om. nocte.

March 22nd.—The "jumping" of the heart is
almost gone, the breath is better, and she rests
better ; continued well till November 5th, 1866,
when, as the cold weather came on she returned,
and, when asked, stated that she had kept pretty
well since her attendance in the spring.

I should not now prescribe arsenic where
hæmoptysis and a feeble heart were present as
prominent symptoms.

CHAPTER VI.

IT is now twelve years since I first became convinced of the value of arsenical preparations in the treatment of certain forms of asthma, and during that period I have never seen harm of any kind from the careful employment of this medicine. The remedy is not new, for A.D. 54 Dioscorides used the sulphuret of arsenic in the treatment of difficult breathing. Arsenic, like sulphur, probably acts by correcting some morbid diathesis in the blood. Arsenic also seems to me to possess some special power in influencing the pneumogastric

G

nerve. Recently I have had under my observation a mother and daughter, the first suffering severely with irritative dyspepsia and vomiting, the second with bad attacks of spasmodic
asthma. In each case the relief obtained from
the use of one drop of Fowler's solution three
times a day was most decided, far surpassing
that from all the numerous medicines previously tried. It seems here reasonable to
suppose that in each case the pneumogastric
nerve was in a state of irritation ; in the
daughter the irritation showed itself in the
pulmonary branches of the nerve, in the mother
in the gastric branches. The same medicine
proved curative to both patients.

To explain the nature of this undue irritability of the pneumogastric nerve seems impossible, but the fact continually comes before
us in practice. One person gets violent dyspepsia, is in fact poisoned if he partakes of
certain articles of food, that to most others are
harmless ; a second individual gets a stoppage
of his breath and spasm at the chest if he

inhales the smell of hay, of linseed meal, or of ipecacuanha powder; substances the odour of which is without effect on most of mankind. In these cases the pneumogastric is poisoned at its pulmonary, rather than at its gastric, extremities.

It will be observed that, in Case VII. phosphorus, in the form of the hypophosphite of soda, did good after arsenic had failed.

The hypophosphites of soda, potash, and lime, are salts that I have long used with advantage in many forms of pulmonary disease. When properly prepared these salts are so rich in phosphorus that they burn when heated on a spatula in the flame of a lamp; they are very soluble salts, and rarely disagree with the stomach, though sometimes a good deal of flatulence is complained of shortly after taking a dose of the hypophosphite.

The hypophosphite salts are preferable to arsenic in cases of asthma, with tendency to bronchitic complications and congestion of lung. The following case illustrates this :—

*Asthmatic attacks at night, with intensely sus-
ceptible chest. Cure by the hypophosphite of
lime.*

CASE VIII.—Ann G., living at Peckham, æt.
42, seen May 20th, 1867. She has been ill
one month with severe cough and frothy expectoration ; at night she is seized with attacks
of asthma, with spasmodic pain across lower
part of chest. She is much worse if it be at
all wet, and one night, on its coming on to rain,
she was at once woke up from her sleep and
obliged to have the fire lighted before the
breathing was at all relieved.

The chest is resonant, and bronchitic *râles*
are audible on both sides.

> ℞ Calcis hypophosphit., gr. v.;
> Aq. menth, pip. ʒj., m. t. d. s.
> Pil. conii., co. gr. v. om. nocte.

Tincture of iodine applied to the chest.

In a fortnight the relief to the breathing was
very decided ; she began then to take quinine.
In a week more the susceptibility of the chest
was greatly diminished, and all signs of bronchitis had entirely vanished.

This is one, as an example, of a class of
cases of very susceptible chest, associated with
more or less true bronchitis; though the difficulty of breathing and asthma is out of all
proportion to the amount of bronchitis present

in the lungs. The hypophosphites of soda, potash, and lime, may often be given with great advantage in these cases, and I believe these salts act partly, by their invigorating effect, on the nervous system.

At times phosphorus, gr. one-fortieth, with sufficient solid fat to make a small pill, or phosphorated oil in one of Tisy's capsules, will answer better than the hypophosphite salts in relieving the dyspnœa.

In the case of a lady, æt. 43 years, who, in consequence of a severe cold, had got chronic bronchitis of eighteen months' duration, with very bad attacks of nocturnal asthma, I tried stramonium, arsenic, mercury, and iodide of potassium without in any way relieving the dyspnœa; and after between two and three months of treatment to very little purpose, I tried the phosphorus pill, gr. one-fortieth, three times daily. After a short time the relief obtained was decided, and for a while, indeed, I thought the patient was cured, but I hear that recently, while away from town, she has had rather a bad relapse.

Sulphur is another medicine valuable in the treatment of spasmodic asthma. It was suggested years ago by Duclos, of France, that asthma was a manifestation in the air tubes of a herpetic diathesis, the varieties of asthma corresponding with various forms of skin disease. On this hypothesis Duclos placed much reliance on arsenic and sulphur as remedies for asthma.

That asthma, in its spasmodic form, often alternates with some chronic skin disease is a point that can be proved by numerous instances. One I have already mentioned, and Case XI. is another illustration. A third I call to mind in a little girl who had well-marked spasmodic asthma following on the cure of a troublesome skin eruption (psoriasis I believe) by Mr. Startin.

Hypophosphite of soda, with iron and a change of locality, appeared to cure this child completely; and I may here mention incidentally that phosphorus and the hypophosphites have proved good medicines in my hands in more than one case of psoriasis of the skin, and in many cases of asthma their curative power has been very decided.

Sulphur is best employed in the form of some

of the sulphur waters found at Harrogate, in Yorkshire, and at Amélie les Bains, in the south-west of France. These waters must be employed only when inflammatory action is quiet, and the warm and mild climate of Amélie will tend greatly to check any bronchitic irritation of the chest, and so prepare the way for the use of the waters.

The hot sulphur springs of Amélie, used in vapour bath and by inhalation, have proved eminently curative in cases of asthma due to sudden suppression of habitual perspiration of the feet.

Another thermal sulphur station of the Pyrenees is found at Cauterets. The sulphur existing in the form of the sulphide of sodium, together with chloride of sodium, silica, and organic matter.

The water of the Raillère spring, at a short distance from Cauterets, enjoys an increasing reputation for the cure of chronic laryngitis and pharyngitis, and especially is this water praised for cases of humid asthma.

If there be any tendency to blood spitting,

the cool and bracing air of Cauterets is preferable to the milder and more sedative climates
of Amélie and Eaux Bonnes.

I have observed some inveterate cases of
asthma to be associated with chronic pharyngitis and laryngitis, the follicles of the tonsils
and pharynx being swelled and irritable ; often
I believe this affection is a true tonsillar herpes,
and in these cases sulphur is one of the best
medicines that can be employed.

When circumstances prevent the patient from
resorting to any of the sulphur springs, we may
try the effect of administering the sulphur in
powder, or as the confection of sulphur of the
B.P. Well-washed sublimed sulphur is generally preferable to the precipitated sulphur, and
it may be given in doses of from five to ten
grains night and morning. with an equal quantity of heavy carbonate of magnesia mixed in
milk.

The oleum sulphuratum, or balsam of sulphur
of the Ph. Lond., 1824, is made by dissolving
one part of sublimed sulphur in eight parts of
olive oil, and is a brown viscid substance with
a most unpleasant smell, the dose is forty to

fifty drops, and it has proved a good remedy to my knowledge in some forms of asthma.

Another preparation of sulphur that I have found serviceable is the sulphurated potash of the B.P. This salt may be given in the form of an alcoholic solution or tincture, or as a pill, containing one or two grains to the dose. Like the balsam of sulphur, the pills have a disgusting smell, but this may be obviated by making them up with some powdered cinnamon and a drop or two of the oil of anise, this last very completely overcomes the odour of the sulphur in the pill.

While the action of preparations of sulphur phosphorus, and arsenic in cases of asthma is often strikingly curative, yet there are plenty of cases where these medicines fail entirely, though the case may be one of pure uncomplicated, spasmodic asthma.

This class of cases must be dealt with on general principles, the object of treatment being to allay irritation of the nervous system and to invigorate the same by means of nerve tonics.

Where the tendency to asthma is due to

rheumatism, the patient being invariably worse in damp weather, the iodide of potassium or ammonium combined with the carbonate of ammonia may be given with confidence. Camphor water or plain water is generally the best vehicle for the administration of these salts, but I have given them sometimes in the infusion of senega, and certainly have found the combination efficacious, though very unpleasant to the taste.

Occasionally the bromide of ammonium succeeds better than the iodide; either salt may be given in a commencing dose of five grains.

Among other medicines at times useful in asthma are: zinc in the form of the oxide and sulphate, silver as nitrate and oxide, and the carbonate and sub-nitrate of bismuth. To lay down precise rules for the administration of these drugs is not easy. Nervous irritability of the system and want of sleep at night would lead one to select zinc; and I usually give the oxide in a pill with ext. hyoscyami —of each, two grains.

The opportunity for using the oxide of silver in dose of a half to one grain appears when there is tendency to gastric irritation, and to very sudden invasion of the asthmatic attack.

The action of bismuth, I believe, is confined to the stomach ; and in cases where an empty and irritable stomach appears the cause of asthmatic attacks, the subnitrate of bismuth may be given in a dose of five to fifteen grains half an hour before a meal.

The mineral acids, and especially the phosphoric acid, are useful in the general treatment of asthma, and so are such tonics as quinine, strychnine, and nux vomica. In those cases where prolongation of the expiration is a marked symptom, the tincture of nux vomica in doses of three to ten drops, or the liquor strychniæ, in doses of three to five drops, will be found admirable medicines, and may very advantageously, in many cases, be combined with some of the preparations of iron.

The two following cases illustrate what has been said :—

A case of asthma, with rheumatoid affection, cured by iodide of potassium.

CASE IX.—William P——, an elderly man, has long suffered with what he calls rheumatic gout affecting the smaller joints, and, in May, 1865, he came under my care at Victoria Park Hospital for attacks of dyspnœa of extreme severity, together with a cough, attended with expectoration, sometimes clear and frothy, at other times yellow and thick. No signs of structural change to be detected in heart or lungs.

The treatment here was very simple, and yet remarkably successful.

It appears that he got a mixture of—

> Potass nitrat.,
> Pot. iodid., āā, gr. v.
> Aq. menth. pip., ʒj., t. d. s.

and this after a fortnight was followed by a chalybeate tonic.

In six weeks the man was discharged cured, and a month or two after wrote a note spontaneously, to express his satisfaction at the immunity from asthma, as well as from any fresh gouty attacks, which he now enjoyed. No expectorants were used in this case, the treatment being mainly directed at the diathetic state.

About six months ago I had under my care, at the West London Hospital, a man who had most severe attacks of nocturnal asthma; his general health was good, he had not much cough, but the asthmatic configuration of chest was marked with some slight evidence of a rheumatic diathesis. I prescribed for him stramonuim, ipecacuanha, conium, and one or two other medicines without the least benefit.

One day in my absence, the house surgeon, Mr. Hill, ordered this man a mixture with iodide of potassium ; and he told me he never had anything before that gave him such relief, he took the mixture for some time, and was discharged greatly relieved.

The following case illustrates beneficial treatment from relieving gastric disturbance and flatulence by charcoal.

Very obstinate asthma.—Failure of several remedies—Eventually much good from the use of acacia charcoal.

CASE X.—This was the case of Mr. O——— who, in consequence of severe asthma of two years' standing, came from Wales to London for advice. Before coming under my hands, he had already been treated by two eminent London practitioners without deriving benefit.

He was about 50 years of age, and after his meals and very often at night he was attacked by fits of asthma, that held him fixed as in a vice ; his face became almost livid with congestion, and the sweat poured off him. Very hot brandy and water and tobacco-smoke after a while relieved him, and the asthma passed off with cough and expectoration.

No organic disease of heart or of lungs could be detected.

To detail all the treatment that this patient underwent would be a very long affair; while in the country he was salivated with decidedly evil effect, and after he came under my notice in London I tried an immense variety of medicines—such as arsenic, nitrate of silver, iodide of potassium, ipecacuanha, &c.—without any benefit whatever.

Eventually good came from the use of pills of ext. nux vomica and the ferrum redactum, but that which really did obtain some easy and undisturbed nights for the patient seemed to be the use, two hours after meals, of powders of the acacia charcoal; from these he got much relief, but I cannot say that to my knowledge he was quite cured.

Hereditary asthma in a brother and sister.—Co-existence of skin affection.—Partial relief from treatment.

CASE XI.—The following case, already casually alluded to, illustrates well the supervention of bad hereditary asthma.

Henry B——, a clerk, æt. 16, living in Essex, came for advice to Victoria Park Hospital, September 21st, 1865. He is a healthy-looking youth, and he complains of severe attacks of spasmodic asthma. States that his father had asthma for thirty-six years, and he has a sister a few years older than himself who has been asthmatical for six years. Mother is free from all sign of the complaint.

Patient first began to be affected with asthma when 13 years of age ; the attacks usually come on about seven in the evening ; he has them also in the night.

For an hour before the attack there is much tightness about the chest, and a feeling as if the chest would burst. He has fits of violent shaking cough, but never much expectoration.

He is always much worse in close, thundery weather ; he cannot at such times remain in bed with comfort.

Tongue is clean and appetite good, but he never touches butcher's meat, as he cannot swallow it ; eats much bacon. The throat, when examined, looks healthy except that the palatine arch on the left side seems more ample than that on the right.

The action of the heart is feeble, but regular. Note is made of prolonged expiration on both sides.

This patient received a mixture containing some of the tr. nux vomica, with dilute phosphoric acid ; and, while taking it, he thought there was less of the constrictive pain about the chest.

In October, as he drew attention to a pustular eruption about face and neck, he was ordered some of the liquor arsenicalis ; and after fourteen days this was changed to a mixture containing three grains of hypophosphite of potash three times in the day, and pil. conii co., five grains, every night.   Under this last medicine he improved, so that he had but two attacks of asthma during the week. At the same time the cutaneous irritation subsided, and he was greatly relieved.

He remained in comfort till some wet weather set in, early in November, then his asthma came on as bad as ever again, and he had six or eight bad attacks in a week.   During these seizures the distention of the chest was so great as almost to burst his clothes open.   The chest in the intervals was extra-resonant, its expansion free, expiration very prolonged, and no *râle* or rhonchal sound could then be heard anywhere.

A pill of extr. stramonii, gr. $\frac{1}{2}$, was now given every night, and he was advised to inhale one or two of the cigarettes de Joy every day.

In February, 1866, this patient suffered severely, his asthma taking him at all times, obliging him to hurry out of church and get to a warm room, where his breath seemed easier. At this time a pill of the ext. belladonna was tried at night, but from it no sort of relief was obtained; indeed, he thought he was worse on the nights when he took this pill.

An important feature in this case was a great tendency to constipation of the bowels, and an appetite that at times was voracious for such things as he could eat; and he seemed to prefer the asthma to the strict dietary that I constantly urged upon him.   I was the more anxious as to the diet from observing that the worst attacks usually occurred on Sunday, when he was at home in the country, and took a good dinner of bacon.

I still see this patient now and then, but, after trying a variety of remedies, we have come to the conclusion that the attacks are best kept in abeyance by attention to the diet and to the digestive functions, and by the use of the cigarettes de Joy. There seems no sign of the approach of any organic disease, and the youth continues his employment to satisfaction.

This young man's sister had dry asthma, with well-marked psoriasis of the skin, and in her case the liquor arsenicalis was of great service. Were the first patient in a condition of life to do such a thing, I should urge, as his best hope of cure, a visit to the climate and waters of Amélie les Bains.

CHAPTER VII.

SPASMODIC asthma, though in the first instance, as we have shown in the preceding pages, a purely nervous affection, will, if unrelieved, produce sooner or later actual disease and structural change, not only in the lungs, but also in the heart, and thus very serious and often incurable evils accumulate upon the unfortunate patient.

It is, as has been already stated, when asthma begins to manifest itself on those who are somewhat advanced in life that these effects are most certainly and most rapidly developed ; hence, when a patient over forty years old begins to be troubled with asthma, with or without catarrh, it is of the greatest consequence that all proper means should be taken to cure the complaint as fast as possible, or it will probably soon cause cardiac dilatation and irregularity; and congestions of the lungs, liver, and brain, will appear as very serious features in the aspect of the case.

Where the asthma begins its attacks during youth the system becomes much more tolerant of the strain and perturbation to which it is subjected, and it is a common thing to find aged asthmatics who have been harassed by the complaint quite from an early age, and who, with the exception of some chronic bronchitis and emphysema of the lung, seem but little damaged.

In the case of a gentleman sixty years old, whom I saw for Dr. Salter in 1869, asthma had become developed during youth, and was now after some thirty years, complicated with bronchitis and some emphysema of the lung.

Advice in this case was sought, on account
of the severe asthmatic paroxysms, and when
free from these the patient's life was one likely
to last for many years.

Recently I have had under my care a man,
aged twenty-seven, liable to most severe asthmatic fits, which are, however, immensely relieved by the inhalation of a few drops of
nitrite of amyl.   The history of his case is
interesting, and runs briefly as follows :—

There is no hereditary tendency in the family
to asthma, gout, or skin disease, and the patient had good health till he was twenty years
old ; he then noticed that after a fit of laughing
he could not get his breath asthmatic spasm
with contracted lung coming on as a result of
violent expiratory effort ; and these fits by
degrees became common at night, or rather
towards early dawn.   At first he had no cough,
but in the course of a year or two a violent
cough with frothy expectoration was added to
his other troubles, and thus the case became
one of complicated bronchitic asthma.

Examining this patient's chest during one of

his worst paroxysms, I counted his respirations as many as 60 in the minute; expiration was much prolonged all over chest, and with the imperfect short inspiration one heard a faint sound of liquid *râle*, which a full inspiration would have brought out in much abundance.

The use of Slade's cigarettes and a mixture of conium with ipecacuanha was of considerable service in this case.

Atmospheric conditions have much influence in causing spasmodic asthma to become complicated with bronchitis. The gentleman whom I saw for Dr. Salter had always lived in a very damp locality, and the last named patient was a man whose dwelling was by the river at Poplar.

The supervention of fits of asthma in a youth, in whose family gout is hereditary, at a time of life when it was usual for this last-named disease to make its first appearance, gives every prospect of a very troublesome though not dangerous form of asthma; and if, when the asthma is fairly set in, the patient rather rapidly should increase in bulk and become stout, another sign is shown of the tendency of the asthma to settle and be confirmed in the system.

We may feel convinced that the pulmonary organs are beginning to suffer damage from protracted asthma when we observe that there is no longer complete freedom from all breath difficulty in the intervals between the fits of severe dyspnœa. The patient is always more or less short breathed, but especially bad in the morning when he rises and begins to move about, and cough and persistent expectoration become more and more annoying. The originally dry asthma will thus become quite of the moist or humoral character, the susceptibility of the chest to cold increases, and the expectoration after a while becomes sometimes frothy, sometimes purulent, under the influence of attacks of bronchitic inflammation.

Gradually the lung tissue loses its elasticity, and the lungs are not sufficiently emptied of air in expiration; the chest movement is therefore small in the way of direct expansion. The chest may be bulged and barrel-like, with an up and down, rather than expansive

motion, in respiration, or it may be flattened
from atrophous emphysema of the lung. The
former state is, in asthmatics, the most common,
and usually indicates a certain degree of
emphysema ; but it is a mistake in asthmatic
cases to infer a high degree of emphysema to
exist merely because of the barrel-like form of
the thorax. On percussion, the chest is extra
resonant and drummy, and in large-lunged
emphysema it may not be easy to make out
the area of cardiac dulness, in consequence of
the heart being overlaid by resonant emphysematous lung.

It is well to note that, as Dr. Walshe has
stated, at page 487 of the second edition of
his work on the lungs, this condition of over-
distention of the lung can be so far improved
by treatment that the area of the heart's super-
ficial dulness can be demonstrably increased.
This fact should be borne in mind, or other-
wise a very careful examination of the heart,
proving such increase of the cardiac dulness,
may lead to the erroneous idea that we have
demonstrated enlargement of the heart instead

of diminution of the lung, and we may be prophesying evil at the very time when we are doing unmistakable good by our treatment. In atrophous, small-lunged, senile emphysema, the cardiac dulness is usually plainly enough made out.

When the face becomes congested, and the jugular veins swollen, the urine loaded with lithates, and the ankles œdematous, then probably it will be found that the right side of the heart is becoming enlarged, and the case becomes one of very grave aspect.

Such is a short outline of some of the symptoms by which we may infer that a case of asthma is becoming more or less complicated with actual structural disease, and we must arrange our prognosis according to the degree in which these symptoms exist, and the way in which they progress.

A certain amount of emphysema of the lung is nearly always found associated with asthma, and, indeed, the emphysema being hereditary, is often, as a congenital infirmity, at the bottom of cases of asthma met with in young children,

and which cannot be traced to any attack of
bronchitis or whooping-cough. Here the emphysema is the cause, not the effect, of the difficult
respiration. In those other cases where the
primary disease is purely nervous in its character, emphysema with dilatation of the air-
vesicles of the lung is gradually brought about
by the excess of respiratory effort, and is pretty
uniformly observed in both lungs.

By degrees, after the emphysema has attained
some extent and existed for some time, we get
atrophic changes produced in the lungs. The
nutrition of the air-cells suffers from insufficient
supply of blood, because, as M. Pousseuille
has shown, with excessive inflation of the lung
a less quantity of fluid passes through the
capillaries in a given time; the cell walls, therefore, become granular looking, fatty, lose their
natural elasticity, and fail progressively in function (*a*).

The lung failing in nutrition and power be-

(*a*) I would refer the reader to an admirable paper on these
points, by Dr. Hensley, in the St. Bartholomew's Reports,
Vol. III.

comes increasingly liable to attacks of bronchitis and congestion; hence we usually find
more or less of chronic bronchitis going along
with emphysema, though, in the first instance,
the emphysema is evolved without any bronchitis of necessity being present.

The majority of asthmatics who come under
treatment present instances of asthma complicated with emphysema and chronic bronchitis,
and when these conditions have for some time
existed in a severe and aggravated form we
get a class of cases of organic or complicated
asthma, presenting features and symptoms
different to those we meet with in spasmodic
asthma, and requiring some modification in
our method of treatment.

These are the cases that have been already
alluded to, where the difficulty in the breathing
is presumed to be of a paralytic rather than of
a spasmodic nature. The labour with these
patients is in *expiration;* they cannot, to quote
the words of a veteran member of the medical
profession lately under my care for this kind of
asthma, " get the air out of the chest."

The nervous irritability is exhausted by repeated attacks of spasm, and verging on paralysis, and though this be not a very promising
aspect of affairs, yet it is certain that much good
can be done, and relief afforded in these cases
without any very complicated process of medication.

I believe the use of sedatives in these cases
is very limited ; opiates indeed should be altogether avoided as harmful, and the medicines
called expectorants—such as squills, senega, and
ammoniacum—do little else than disturb and
nauseate the stomach, without rendering us
much help to relieve the chest.   I have thought
sometimes that the tincture of lobelia, in doses
of thirty to sixty drops, the tincture of benzoin,
and the tincture of larch bark, have done temporary good where there has been a good deal
of puriform expectoration ; but I have never
seen anything like the permanent good effect
from any of the above-named remedies that I
have seen come of a careful use of some of the
ordinary well-known tonics ; all expectorant
remedies being banished from the field of action

at the same time. That which, from its occurring more than once, has impressed me as remarkable, is the circumstance that some of the
patients of the class above described have a
strong prejudice against taking tonics. An old
gentleman who, under the belief that his asthma
was due to suppressed gout, and who was often
told that he "ought to have the gout," and had
been thoroughly drenched with a variety of al-
caline waters to no purpose, told me that whatever he took it must not be a tonic. The medicine he had, and the only medicine that he
declared had ever done him good, was the
tincture of nux vomica with dilute phosphoric
acid, and we never entered upon any discussion
again as to whether tonics were suitable or not.

It strikes me as very probable that this aversion of the emphysematous asthmatic to the use
of tonics has its foundation in the circumstance
of these remedies having been inopportunely or
prematurely, and perhaps rather pertinaciously,
tried at some earlier period in the case when
the indications were rather in favour of the use
of anti-spasmodics alone ; or at a time when some

passing attack of true bronchitic inflammation might have required the temporary use of salines or expectorants.

It is when there is absence of true inflammation, and when expectoration and difficult breathing seem always to be worse as the patient gets weaker, that expectorants are of so little service, while bark, iron, and quinine come in as invaluble remedies permanently to benefit the dyspnœa by invigorating the general system.

When we consider further what the condition of the respiratory organs appears to be in these cases of old standing complicated asthma, we shall see why tonics and remedies likely to improve nutrition are so strongly indicated.

The chest is in a constant state of over-distention, and the lungs themselves are over-full of air, just as they are when they are paralysed by section of the vagus nerve, and there seems good reason to think that in some of these cases it is insufficient innervation of the lungs that is the cause of the dyspnœa rather than any great amount of emphysema of the lung substance. I have for a long time practically

felt that we must recognise this paralytic form
of asthma with very difficult expiration, as distinct from spasmodic asthma with closed lungs,
and it is with much satisfaction I observe that
both Dr. Walshe and Dr. Fuller recognise the
same distinction. That this form of asthma may
be a true paralysis is proved by Dr. Fuller, who
has traced some of these cases after death and
found very trifling emphysema of the lungs,
though during life the dyspnœa had been excessive. " Fuller on the Lungs," second edition,
p. 375-6. In these cases of dyspnœa the movement of the lower part of the chest-walls and
especially of the diaphragm should be closely
watched.

In one of the most highly developed instances
that I ever beheld of pulmonary emphysema of,
as I judged, atrophous kind, resulting from
severe asthma of thirty years' duration, the
patient remarked on the relief that he derived
from the process of percussion over his chest.
The thumping with the fingers over the chest
seemed to dislodge the stagnant air from the
lungs, and so had a reviving effect on the

patient. These are the cases that appear to get good from breathing a condensed and concentrated atmosphere in a chamber built for the purpose. Though there is much that is discouraging in the prospect of attempting to treat the case of one, the air cells of whose lungs are losing their natural elasticity and undergoing a process of degeneration, yet we must recollect that it is impossible to obtain absolutely certain evidence that real degeneration of tissue has set in, and in a large number of these cases of paralytic and emphysematous asthma the real and permanent good that can be done with the tincture of nux vomica, and with very small doses of strychnia, is unmistakably great. The tincture may be given in doses of from three to eight, or ten drops, and the liquor strychniæ of the British Pharmacopœia in doses of two to five drops.

My own plan is to keep to very small doses administered in a simple medium, such as mint water; and given thus carefully and watchfully I have never seen the slightest evil effect produced, though from what I have been told by

one of the most careful and judicious prescribers
in London, I feel bound to urge great caution
and great watchfulness when using strychnine
itself, even in so small a dose as 1-30th of a
grain persistently; further, as a precautionary
measure, it is well so to arrange the prescription
that there can never be more than half a grain
of strychnine in the house at once.

Less efficacious than nux vomica and strychnine comes quinine, and this remedy when given
to an asthmatic should be dissolved in phosphoric or nitric acid. Given thus, it may be set
down as often a very useful medicine.

Iron is, as a tonic, especially valuable, and
yet often the patients fear to take it, saying it
will increase the cough. It rarely does this, and
the tincture of the perchloride of iron, the sulphate of iron, and the citrate of iron, are all very
valuable preparations, and go well with strychnine or with quinine. The sulphate or perchloride of iron may be given with some of the
sulphate of magnesia or soda in cases where the
liver and bowels are sluggish in action.

In the cases of those who are markedly worse

when there is much damp about, the iodide of potassium is worth a trial; and given with some ammonia and citrate of iron it forms a combination of considerable service.

The preparations of arsenic, so useful in the dry forms of asthma, are quite second to nux vomica, iron, and mineral acids, in the treatment of humoral asthma; when, however, we suspect the asthma to be connected with some morbid diathesis, arsenic and also sulphur are quite worthy of a fair trial.

It happens not unfrequently that in these cases of complicated asthma there are at night attacks of spasm of the lungs—these must be met by those remedies already mentioned, such as ether, datura tatura, and medicated inhalations. Sedatives at night do not interfere with other remedies during the day, but it is well not to be in too great a hurry to resort to them, for it is not uncommon to find such a medicine as nux vomica overcome spasm and give the patient a better night's rest than anything else that has ever been tried in the way of antispasmodic or sedative.

I

I have tried warm medicated inhalations in some of these cases of emphysematous asthma, but unless the complaint be due to irritative bronchitis they do not do much good, and many patients say they seem to relax and weaken the lungs. Creasote and the oil of pine seem the most promising substances for use in the inhaler.

The inhalation of compressed air, and its remedial power in asthma, with emphysematous lungs, has already been mentioned more than once. Though I cannot speak from any great personal observation or experience, yet I feel bound to respect the evidence of those who speak so favourably of this form of inhalation in the treatment of asthma.

The condensed atmosphere must of necessity carry a proportionately larger amount of oxygen into the chest, and so relieves the distress due to the imperfect aëration of the blood in the lungs; the craving and hunger of the system for more oxygen is therefore relieved by filling the lungs with a condensed atmosphere.

The fact that a condensed atmosphere keeps up the necessary supply of oxygen longer than one of ordinary tension, was observed years ago by Brunel when engaged in making the Thames Tunnel. This great engineer having occasion, at times, to descend under water in a diving bell, and now and then, in order to examine specially certain points in the works, quitting the bell for the water itself, found that he could remain under water, without serious distress, for a length of time that excited the alarm of his companions in the bell ; this power was attributed to the fact of the lungs being inflated with the atmosphere of the bell, which was denser and richer in oxygen than that at the water's surface (*a*).

Another remedial agent in emphysematous asthma, that has had its warm advocates, is electricity; and here, as in a host of other affections, this agent has been tried in the most empirical way, and on the vague hypothesis that asthma, being a nervous disease, is sure to be relieved by any power that acts in any way

(*a*) In Chap. IX. see effect of compressed air on the heart and blood vessels, with places where this treatment is employed.

on the nerves, especially if these be tending to a paralytic state.   I have little to offer from my own experience of the use of electricity in asthma, but I can understand that the continuous current, from one of Pulvermacher's chains, or any other source, might be of use in overcoming spasm.   To the experience of my friend Dr. Althaus I am indebted for the following remarks on the use of galvanism in asthma :—

In true spasmodic asthma not complicated with emphysema or other structural lesions, but purely nervous in its origin, the continuous galvanic current directed to the pneumogastric nerve in the neck, near the carotid artery, appears to be an excellent remedy, which, as yet, has not been fully tried.

The induced current applied to the same nerve is without effect ; any form of electricity applied to the chest-wall is also ineffectual.

The application of the continuous current to the pneumogastric should be very gentle, and continue for not more than two minutes at a time.

Long and strong applications irritate the nerve and excite an asthmatic attack.

The direction of the current should be inverse in cases where the nervous circuit, the irritation of which produces the asthmatic attack, appears to be in the brain ; a gentle application to the head should be combined with that to the pneumogastric nerve.

In these cases of emphysematous asthma, with general debility and absence of inflammation, a dry bracing climate is of the greatest possible service when there is a good deal of cough and expectoration, with languor of the system. In cases of great irritability and spasm of the chest one that is mild and warm is to be preferred.

The food must be light and nutritious, and must be taken in but small quantities at a time, with pale sherry, or weak brandy and water, as the drink that will agree best with the majority of cases. Casual attacks of flatulence and acidity are best met by the use of Belloc's charcoal lozenges, or by sucking a pastille of the Vichy salt, both of which remedies, from their convenient form, can be carried about easily by the patient.

CHAPTER VIII.

Bronchitic asthma, or the dyspnœa of chronic and sub-acute
bronchitis.—Sudden attacks of dyspnœa from obstruction
of a bronchial tube.—Production of dilated bronchial
tubes.—This is a troublesome and often permanent complication.—Treatment of bronchitic asthma.—Curative power
of climate.—Importance of subduing any persistent inflammation.—Use of mercury and other remedies.—Illustrative
cases.

THE object of the present chapter is to offer a
few observations on the asthmatic complications
of chronic and sub-acute bronchitis.

In these cases we have inflammatory action,
plus spasmodic exacerbations, due to irritation of
certain nerves. We see examples of these accessions of severe and dangerous spasm constantly
in cases of laryngitis and croup; there is a true
inflammatory process going on sufficiently dangerous in itself, and from time to time attacks of
spasm in the breathing occur that add greatly

to the immediate danger, and that are best met, not by local depletion or sharp counter-irritation. but by sedative appliances and inhalations.

An individual who may from any cause have become the victim of chronic bronchitis is well known to be liable to attacks of severe breath difficulty in the event of his taking a fresh cold, or in consequence of any sudden change in the weather. The attacks vary in degree, but their symptoms are just those of asthma, and I have always put these cases down in my note-book as cases of *bronchitic asthma:* they may be of a gouty or rheumatic origin, and there may be more or less emphysema of the lungs present; but the most distinctive mark is the origin of the asthma in bronchitis, or some other inflammatory affection of the chest, the result most commonly of cold.

The breathing is always more or less difficult, and alterations of temperature, or of degree of humidity in the air, powerfully, and at once, affect the patient. At night there is often great distress, with sometimes complete inability to lie down in bed ; or else the patient, after lying

for a short time, suddenly has to start up in a
fit of severe dyspnœa and spasm. Expectora·
tion may be scanty or copious, with at times a
little blood, and the sputum itself may vary
greatly, being at one time frothy and almost
clear, at another time, within a few hours, it may
be thick and yellow. These sudden variations
seem to me oftenest noticed in cases of bronchitis complicated with rheumatism.

Sometimes the cough is violent and paroxysmal, and after a burst of coughing there follows a regular fit of asthma, the lungs are
emptied of air by the cough, and remain for a
time in a state of spasmodic contraction.

It should be remembered that it will sometimes happen that a patient (probably one rather
advanced in years) ill with chronic bronchitis
may be seized, without warning, with a sudden
attack of extreme dyspnœa that brings him even
to the verge of suffocation.

These seizures in the sudden manner of their
invasion, and the equally sudden manner in
which they pass off, resemble attacks of spasmodic asthma supervening upon chronic bron-

chitis. They are not, however, attacks purely spasmodic in their nature, but they are in very many instance certainly due to collapse of a portion of lung from plugging up of the air-tube which leads to this portion of collapsed lung.

The obstruction is caused usually by a lump of thickened mucus, like those firm round lumps of mucus that are sometimes expectorated by persons ill with chronic bronchitis, and which I have had brought to me in bottles by patients who were somewhat alarmed at the size and firmness of the ball of mucus which they had coughed up. This ball of mucus forming in an air-tube acts the part of a valve, permitting the egress of air in expiration, but preventing its entry into the lung by inspiration. Thus at last the portion of lung is perfectly emptied of air, and it collapses into one of those condensed masses that were called instances of lobular pneumonia till Dr. Gairdner explained their true nature and mode of production.

In this form of dyspnœa there will be great and marked difficulty in the act of inspiration, while that of expiration is comparatively easy.

When the attack is perfectly developed it will
be found that over the collapsed portion of the
lung there is complete dulness on percussion
and no respiratory sound can be heard, when before probably bronchial *râles* were quite distinct.

These attacks may last from one to twenty-
four hours, and as they pass away the breath
sound will be observed to return and the percussion dulness to subside at the affected part
of the lung.

In a case related to me not long since by
the patient, who is himself a physician, troublesome dyspnœa and discomfort on the left side
of the chest, that had existed for some weeks,
was in no way relieved till the patient coughed
up a round ball of hard mucus. There seems
reason to believe that this, by rendering a portion of the left lung non-expansile, has produced some limited emphysema which still
remains.

The fibrinous casts of the bronchi expectorated in inveterate asthma, as well as in
chronic plastic bronchitis, are familiar to most
observers. When placed in spirit these casts

spread out and look like the roots of some plant. Among a numerous and highly interesting collection of these casts, placed by Dr. Peacock in the Museum of the Victoria Park Hospital, is one rather large fibrinous ramification coughed up by an asthmatic gentleman who is said to have afterwards died of phthisis. The probability is that these fibrinous masses, blocking up portions of the lung, may eventually give rise to breaking down and softening of the pulmonary tissue, just as fibrinous deposits from the blood have been shown to do by Dr. Andrew Clark and Dr. Niemeyer; and thus the patient dies with all the symptoms of softening and excavation of the lung. Some of the best examples of fibrinous expectoration that I have seen have been in cases of asthma with atrophic emphysema of the lungs ; the nutritive tendency of the system tending to fibrosis more than to pus formation. These are the cases where after a while one gets dulness at one apex from fibroid condensation of lung, and at times there follow hæmoptysis, and all the symptoms of gradually advancing phthisis.

There is another pathological state met with often in these cases of bronchitic asthma, associated too with emphysema, and that is dilatation of the bronchial tubes. The presence of dilated bronchial tubes in the chest of a grown-up person is likely to be a permanent evil, and will maintain the tendency to bronchitis and dyspnœa.

Inflammatory action in and around the air-tubes after long continuance leads to exudation of contractile lymph ; which, if on the tissue external to the tube, draws upon and dilates the tube, while at the same time it renders the lung tissue less expansile. When the inspiratory efforts become powerful and strong the tubes are distended more and more, they cannot contract as they are wont to do in health, they yield and stretch under the strain put upon them, secretion stagnates in them in increasing quantity, their tissue becomes weak and degenerate, and dyspnœa increases and remains abiding.

The physical signs of enlarged bronchial tubes are pretty well known, and it is in the infra-mammary regions where these should be especially sought ; here we may find want of expansion, dulness on percussion, occasionally a true "crackpot" note, with hollow bronchial breathing and very prolonged expiration. I have in rare instances of old chronic bronchitis, following on neglected pneumonia, observed true amphoric breathing over the bases of the lungs, apparently due to globular dilatation of the bronchial tubes. This condition was exceedingly well marked in the case of a man under Dr. Risdon Bennett, in Victoria Park Hospital, some years ago. This man had been ill some years previously with pneumonia, and he was sent up from the country to the hospital on account of the bronchitis and asthma which clung to him ; he was somewhat benefited by treatment, but with so much structural change it was impossible to look for more than some relief to the more urgent symptoms.

Provided there be no great structural change in the way of dilated air-tubes, emphysematous lungs, or enlarged heart, we may look for very satisfactory results from treatment in these cases of bronchitic asthma.

I suppose there is no remedy so radically curative as climate for these cases. I have seen cases of bronchitis with much irritation of the chest, scanty secretion, and tendency to spasmodic difficulty in the breathing, improve speedily, progressively, and permanently at such places as Hastings, Ventnor, and Bournemouth. My own observation and experience of climates for bronchitic asthma is limited mainly to these places, as I find them to succeed so well; but there are other well-known resorts possessing a similar mild sedative air, such as Torquay, Sidmouth, and Penzance, which would do well for the bronchitic invalid, though they are not good for one who is far gone in pulmonary consumption, save for the purposes of promoting a euthanasia.

Cases with highly-developed emphysema, languor of system and profuse secretion, must avoid all places that are of a sedative and relaxing nature, and seek some of the dry bracing places like Harrowgate or Malvern inland, and Scarborough, Brighton, Margate, or Cromer, on the sea coast.

The point wherein the medicinal treatment of these cases of bronchitic asthma, in a measure, differs from that of emphysematous asthma is that we have a smouldering kind of low inflammatory action as the root of the mischief; and as we often have to deal with thickenings and exudations of inflammatory origin, it is here that some of the absorbent remedies, such as mercury, the iodides, and the alkalies, come in most happily before we resort to the more tonic class of medicines.

The clearing off of inflammation, and of the products of inflammation, I regard as a most important point in the curative treatment of cases of bronchitic asthma, and for this purpose we have among our drugs the various preparations of mercury which are here most valuable. I may say that I have never in any case given mercury so as in any way to affect the mouth. The way in which I use it will be easily seen by a perusal of the cases of bronchitic asthma appended to this chapter.

When the bronchitic state of lung is subdued any emphysema which may remain must be treated on the principles already enunciated.

The following are selected from the notes of
a large number of cases of bronchitic asthma ;
they will serve to illustrate those points in the
treatment of the complaint to which attention
has been already drawn.

*Cough and nocturnal dyspnœa, slight benefit from
cod-liver oil and iodide of iron, cured by mercurials.*

CASE XII.—Robert R., æt. 16 years, came
under treatment October 10th, 1865. He is a
pale, light-haired youth, and his complaint is of
cough, and much thick yellow expectoration
consequent on neglected cold. He has never
raised any blood, the tongue is clean, tonsils
very large, chest is resonant, but some few crepi-
tating sounds are heard in upper part of left
lung. Pulse 120.

Till October 26th he was treated with cod-
liver oil and iodide of iron, and at first he
improved on these medicines; but on October
26th he seemed to have taken some fresh cold,
for the cough was very severe at night, and
after the fits of cough he had asthmatic wheezing often so loud as to be audible in the next
room. Pulse 120, bronchitic sounds to limited
extent in left lung; he does not himself consider
that he has improved on the treatment thus far.

For the next fortnight he took every night a
pill of pulv. scillæ et pil. hydrarg., of each two
grains; he continued cod-liver oil and took

some nitrate of potash and vin. ipecac. with mucilage, three times daily.

November 8th.—Rest much better, much less spit, not near so much cough, breath easy, tongue clean, pulse still keeps up. To take pil. conii. co., five grains, in place of pil. hydrarg.

November 23rd.—He had some iodide of ammonium in a mixture, and on December 14th he was discharged free from cough, and only complaining of dyspnœa on exertion; further than this the note does not go, for I did not then know I should ever publish the case.

The point of interest in this case was the absence of all real improvement till the man got the small doses of mercury. I suspected strongly that the left lung was about to become tubercular, but have had no reason to believe that it ever did become so.

That paroxysmal asthma, of very violent nature, in young people is, at times, a sign of commencing miliary tubercles in the lungs, is a point on which we have certain evidence from recorded cases and *post-mortem* examinations.

Dyspnœa due solely to chronic bronchitis and soon removed by mercurials.

Case XIII.—Henry W., æt. 45 years, seen October 7th, 1867. For some months has had

K

severe cough night and day, with thick expectoration. At night much difficulty in the breathing and profuse sweating.   Pulse 80; face pale. Chest resonant; respiration generally feeble, with some sonorous and sibilant rhonchus.

R Pil. Hydrarg.
    Pulv. scillæ, āā, gr. ij. pil. om. nocte.

R Vin. ipecac., ℳ viij.
    Tr. opii., ℳ iij.
    Potass nitrat., gr. v.
    Mist. acac., ʒj , m. t. d. s.

He had no other medicine, and on October 28th he was let go, describing himself as quite well, able to sleep quietly at night, and free from cough. The cure in this instance was so complete, that the man desired to present me with an article of his manufacture as a token of his satisfaction.

CASE XIV.—Mrs. R., æt. about 40, seen September, 1872.   For thelast two months has had violent cough with frothy expectoration.   At night the difficulty of breathing is extreme, and she has to be propped up in bed with pillows.

No emaciation ; pulse 100 ; face pale ; rather anxious looking ; eyes somewhat suffused ; tongue furred behind.

Appetite not good ; is very careful and abstemious in her manner of living.

She has already taken much medicine, but the severe attacks of spasmodic dyspnœa at night grow worse.

The chest is resonant ; its movement is up and down rather than a true expansion.   Sonorous *râles* are heard over both lungs, with very prolonged expiration.

Sedative inhalations were ordered, and a mixture of hypophosphite of soda with carbonate of ammonia.

Slight improvement took place in the course of the next two weeks.

September 22nd.—I saw her in consequence of a fresh cold, and found the dyspnœa extreme. Pulse 100; moist *râles* over both lungs. A pill was ordered as follows to be taken every night:

> ℞ Pil. Hydrarg., gr. ij.
> Pulv. Ipecac., gr. j.
> Ext. Conii., gr. ij.   M.,

and a mixture of carbonate of ammonium with iodide of potassium.

In eight days' time the report sent was, " Progressing rapidly towards recovery," and she did recover of this attack, though the chest remains exceedingly susceptible to any change of temperature.

The following cases illustrate the development of bronchitic and spasmodic asthma in early childhood.

Bronchitic asthma in a child.   Slight relief from treatment.

CASE XV.—Christian S., æt. 10 years, not thin or emaciated, and of a healthy family; has suffered during the last three years with severe attacks of dyspnœa in winter and summer alike.

Hard cough night and morning and "rears up" at night with the fits of difficult breathing. His mother says he has from birth been weak in the chest.

Pulse 84, tongue clean, pain felt chiefly under sternum. Thorax is extra resonant, a little exertion soon brings on the dyspnœa, and then the upper part of thorax is drawn up and moves but little, while the lower parts and the false ribs open out powerfully in inspiration.

Râles with prolonged expiration noted all over chest ; but decidedly most marked under left clavicle.

Commenced treatment April 16, 1868, thus—

> ℞ Liq. Fowleri, ɱj.,
> Ifst. Calumbæ c Soda ℥ss. t. d. s.
> Pil conii co., gr. ij. om. nocte.

May 7th. -- Has continued the treatment, with the addition of potass. iodid. gr. ij to his mixture, but is not any better ; turns almost black in the face with dyspnœa at times, and has coughed up blood. A mixture was ordered with some of the hypophosphite of potash. Slight amendment followed upon this, and soon after he ceased attending the hospital.

Severe spasmodic asthma with emphysema.

CASE XVI.—Master V. D., æt. 7 years, seen by me August, 1866, in consequence of severe fits of spasmodic asthma, coming on chiefly at night, with lividity of face.

The boy is very intelligent and active, face pale,

some enlargement of cervical glands, chest everywhere fully resonant, sibilant wheezings heard with prolonged expiration. Pulse 86, tongue clean. Any excess of food always brings on the asthma. Suffers with nocturnal incontinence of urine.

This patient has been pretty constantly under my observation up to the present date, and still suffers severely with asthma. At times in damp and cold weather he gets bronchitis, and the asthmatic fits are then more severe, there is now much less lividity during the fit than there used formerly to be.

The extra resonance of the chest, and the very feeble inspiratory murmur with prolonged expiration, render it probable that this case is complicated with emphysema.

An immense variety of medicines were tried in this case, and of these the most valuable were found to be Fowler's solution—belladonna, nitric acid, and iodide of potassium.

Inhalation of a mixture of Verbascum and Stramonium, soaked in a solution of nitre and then dried, served to relieve the paroxysms; and for the same purpose the paper made by Mr. Dowling of Exeter, was of great value. Strong coffee also, I observed, to act well in relieving a severe fit which the young patient had while at the seaside.

In the case of C. H., a little boy, 6 years old, who had fits of mild asthma at night, with incontinence of urine; after failing to do any good with conium and hypophosphite of potash, I at last relieved him very greatly of his asthma, and cured his enuresis by Tinctr. Lyttæ c. Tr. Ferri, of each 5 drops three times daily, in water. In the previous case these medicines had no effect.

In these cases of spasmodic and bronchitic asthma occurring in young children, I believe it to be of much importance to recognize, and as far as possible cure, whatever inflammatory condition there may be going on in the chest. Next, it is of vital importance that the child should be placed in a suitable climate, and be properly cared for in the way of clothing and diet. When these conditions are properly fulfilled, we may reasonably hope to see the disease subside, or become much mitigated in severity by the lapse of time. Without attention to these matters the child will most certainly grow into disease rather than out of it.

CHAPTER IX.

A short account of the effects of asthma on the heart and blood vessels.—Enlargement of the right side of the heart.—Symptoms and signs.—Cardiac dyspnœa.—Means to be employed for relief.—Medicines.—Digitalis.—Salines.—Tonics.—Blood-letting, at times, necessary to relieve the right side of the heart.—Salutary effect of a dry climate.—Effect on the circulation of compressed air.—Reichenhall and its air baths.

ALLUSION has been already made to the extreme smallness of the pulse during a bad paroxysm of asthma, as a sign that there is a stoppage of the circulation through the lungs, causing but a scanty supply of blood to enter the left ventricle and arterial system.

Two circulations are constantly going on in the lungs—the one of air, the other of blood,—and one cannot be checked or arrested without the other participating in such stoppage. In asthma, the aërial circulation being in arrest, the blood circulation suffers in consequence. In heart disease, the blood circulation through the lungs being ·impeded, the aërial circulation suffers consequently, and we get cardiac asthma as the result.

Frequent stoppage of the flow of blood through the lungs, with venous engorgement and stasis, after a while produces dilatation of the right side ·of the heart, and this is the most common cardiac effect of protracted attacks of dyspnœa and asthma. When the heart becomes affected the form of dyspnœa undergoes some modification. Without being periodic, as pure asthma often is, it is irregularly and suddenly paroxysmal, and during these fits there is a look of alarm about the patient, with much gasping and panting. The paroxysm is short, but leaves a good deal of permanent dyspnœa behind with more or less passive bronchitis and tendency to pulmonic congestion. Examination of the chest may show the heart's impulse diffused and readily felt at the epigastrium ; the area of dulness is increased to the right, there is want of tone in the first sound of the heart, the jugular veins are full and prominent, the complexion dusky and more or less livid, signs of congestion of lungs, liver, and stomach appear, the feet swell, the bowels are costive, the urine turbid, and the nights are especially distured.

Such are the signs of an engorged right heart and venous system ; and when they appear in the case of one who is asthmatic they are of evil augury, as showing that the organic complications of the asthma extend beyond the lungs themselves to the heart and circulatory apparatus. The general plan of treatment should be to relieve congestion, and then to try and strengthen the weak and failing structures.

An excellent medicine, in these cases, is found in the infusion and tincture of digitalis. For years I have used these preparations with most satisfactory results, and never yet saw any danger arise from the asserted cumulative action of the drug, though I must confess to having heard of some mishaps when the digitalis has been persevered with in full dose for a long time.

From two to four drachms of the infusion, or five to twenty drops of the tincture, with some nitrate of potash, nitrous ether, and camphor water, is my own standard form, save when I use the pill of powdered digitalis one grain, and powdered squills two grains.

Various saline combinations, sometimes with a diuretic, sometimes with a laxative intent, come in very serviceably to relieve venous congestion, and can be arranged to the judgment of the physician. As soon as there seems to be relief to the more urgent and oppressive symptoms it is well to get in some iron or bark. The iron may be given in a small dose of one grain of the sulphate, or ten drops of the tincture, with sulphate of magnesia, in peppermint water. The bark may be best given with iodide of potassium, and aromatic spirit of ammonia.

It will now and then—when the right heart is much engorged and the oppression in breathing very great—be necessary to draw a little blood. From six to eight ounces taken from the arm relieves occasionally, as nothing else will. Stimulants, so commonly and often so profusely given, merely seem to help the left ventricle to pump the venous system all the more full of blood, while a little relief by the detraction of blood does wonders to restore the balance of the circulation. When I have felt rather timid about opening a vein in the arm, I have applied one or two leeches over the lower part of the sternum, and have reason to speak most favourably of this method.

The heart being in so large a measure influenced by the action of the lungs, we must not forget the importance of a perfectly dry warm climate, and to the power of this as a powerful means of prolonging life I can fully testify, and that, too, when the organic heart mischief was unmistakable.

Speaking of the inhalation of a suitable atmosphere, brings me once again to mention the condensed air-chamber, for it is in cases of dyspnœa, with venous plethora and congestion, where the condensed air claims to be especially curative. At Reichenhall in Bavaria, Montpelier, and Wiesbaden, these air-chambers are to be found at work; and for a full and concise description of the mechanical arrangement of the chamber I must refer the reader to Dr.

Burdon Sanderson's article on "Reichenhall and its Compressed Air Baths," in the *Practitioner* for October, 1868.

The pressure employed in Mr. Mack's Reichenhall Baths is equal to one atmosphere and a half; *i. e.*, about forty-five inches of mercury, or about twenty-two pounds on every square inch of surface. The patient remains in the chamber about an hour and forty minutes; of which time about forty minutes are occupied in gradually and cautiously increasing and diminishing the pressure. The physiological effect of the compressed air bath on the circulation consists in its altering the distribution of the blood, so that while the quantity contained in the veins and auricles of the heart is diminished, that in the ventricles and arteries is increased, and thus the balance of the circulation is restored. Practically it is found that cases of dyspnœa, with old standing emphysema and bronchitis, over-fulness of the venous system, and emptiness and diminished tension of the arterial system, are relieved by the inhalation of the compressed air.

Dr. Vevinot, in his experiments with compressed air at Nice, noted great retardation of pulse and respiration, the former falling as low as eighteen in the minute in one instance ; the secretion of the skin and aërian mucous membrane was at the same time checked, while that of the kidneys was enormously increased.

In the case of workmen employed in building the Mississippi bridge at St. Louis, working in an air chamber, at a pressure of as much as sixty pounds to the square inch, Dr. Bauer observed that many were stricken down with paraplegia, and some died with inflammation of the brain, cord, and membranes.

Trustworthy information, recently obtained from an engineer of much experience among men working in diving bells and cylinders, hardly confirms the statement on page 44.

It appears that all men conscious of any kind of chest weakness, specially of a consumptive nature, learn, by experience, to avoid this kind of labour.

To descend in a bell with anything like a cold or bronchitis about one is described as agony, relieved sometimes by free bleeding from the nose. Work at foundation laying in the air cylinder is more trying than diving bell work, because the pressure is higher, and comes upon one more suddenly. Six minutes in an air cylinder has been known to bring on a profound faint, with blueness of lips, and apparent death, recovery being very protracted.

These points show how powerful is the influence of compressed air on the circulation, and what caution is requisite when employing it therapeutically.

Gradually to increase and diminish the pressure in the bath is most essential, for without care on this point it may happen that a patient who may have felt much relief while in the air-chamber, will experience a most trying reaction, in the way of dyspnœa, after his return into an ordinary atmosphere. In the case of a patient of mine this reaction proved so severe that the bath had to be given up entirely: though, while confined within it, the patient would fall into such a perfect and tranquil sleep as he had not had for many years.

When the apparatus is managed with caution —as it is by the Messrs. Mack at Reichenhall— the treatment seems perfectly safe and free from all risk, and doubtless may sometimes prove a useful method of dealing with cases of protracted and persistent asthma due to chronic bronchitis and emphysema.

CHAPTER X.

I INTRODUCE this as a short supplementary
chapter, for the purpose of entering more fully
into the above named forms of dyspnœa, already
alluded to in the preceding chapters.

Ordinary asthma is a pulmonary or bronchial
spasm, but we may get symptoms closely similar to those of asthma from spasm of the larynx
and closure of the glottis.

An example of this laryngeal asthma is seen
in that nervous affection of young children known
as " Thymic Asthma," " Kopp's," and " Millar's
Asthma," and also as Laryngismus Stridulus;
and before pronouncing a child in its first year
to have congenital asthma, it is as well to see
that the case be not one of laryngismus stridulus.

In laryngismus stridulus, or laryngeal asthma,
the adductor muscles of the vocal cords are
spasmodically contracted, so that they more or
less completely close the laryngeal opening.
The cause of the laryngeal spasm is not more
clear than are the causes of bronchial spasm,
but the disease is well known to be most common in children during the first years of life.
It may be due to teething, to pressure on nerves
of larynx by enlarged glands, or to any other
source of reflex irritation.

In the attack inspiration is noticed to be very
harsh and prolonged with stridor ; and, if the
spasm increases to a complete closure of the
glottis, all respiratory movement ceases, and
suffocation is imminent.

Throughout there is not any fever, but in
very severe cases general convulsions may come
on, with livid face and swelled jugular veins.

Adults sometimes get attacks of laryngeal
spasm and dyspnœa; doubtless often called asthma till the laryngoscope enabled us to ascertain
their true nature.

In the laryngeal spasm of adults the vocal

L

cords, viewed by the laryngoscope, are spasmodically adducted, and so the glottis is closed.
The obvious result of this is to cut off the supply
of air to the lungs. Inspiration becomes long,
laborious, and marked by stridor, while the soft
and yielding parts of the chest wall, at the supraclavicular and intercostal regions fall in and
are depressed in consequence of the non-inflation
of the lung.

Thus we get a case of laryngeal dyspnœa, far
more serious and critical than the dyspnœa of
spasmodic bronchial asthma.

Prolonged inspiration of very high pitch, with
feeble breath sound in lungs, would also occur in
case of tracheal stricture, independently of laryngeal affection.—*See* case of Dr. Morell Mackenzie's
in the Pathological Transactions, 1871, p. 33.

In the *Lancet* of January 23rd, 1864, Sir Duncan
Gibb reported a case of laryngeal and tracheal
obstruction that came under my notice at Victoria Park Hospital. The harsh laryngeal stridor in inspiration was marked while the breath
sounds in chest were feeble, and the supraclavicular spaces fell in during inspiration.

From these symptoms I diagnosed laryngeal

dyspnœa, and Sir Duncan Gibb, who kindly examined the patient, clearly made out the obstruction to be caused by growths impeding the movement of the vocal cords. After death both larynx and trachea were found much obstructed by growths and deposit. In laryngeal dyspnœa expiration is not often prolonged unless the obstruction exist below the glottis. In glottic œdema inspiration is prolonged and hissing; expiration short and easy (Pitha).

Expiratory stridor has been observed by Dr. Fuller in cases where the trachea has been compressed by enlarged bronchial glands. The sign is important in distinguishing these cases from those of true croup. Where expiration and inspiration are alike prolonged and difficult, there probably exists some laryngeal paralysis. This condition of laryngeal paralysis is well illustrated by the following cases :—

CASE XVII.—Mrs. M., æt. 42, has attended at Victoria Park Hospital since 1862, being then under the late Dr. Ingram. She has suffered much from chronic rheumatism, with bronchitis and asthma. Her mother died of asthma, and her father died at the age of 67 of some disease of the chest.

During the autumn of 1869 this patient's breath difficulty increased greatly, and none of the ordinary remedies gave her relief. Inspiration was noted as noisy and difficult, expiration was also very difficult and prolonged. Chest resonance was good, but breath sounds were weak everywhere, as there was but little movement of air in the tubes. Heart sounds normal.

The prolongation of expiration was best observed by auscultation of the larynx.

To see the larynx in the mirror was not easy, but on October 30th it looked to me congested and swollen, with much mucus about it. Subsequent examination satisfied me of something abnormal about the cords, and at my request Dr. Morell Mackenzie very kindly examined the patient with me in March, 1870; and, though there was a good deal of mucus about the throat with congestion and great irritability; yet, when this had been subdued by the use of ice, it was made out that there was paralysis of the abductor and adductor muscles of the left vocal cord, so that this cord remained immoveable, and interchange of air in the chest was a matter of great difficulty.

The attempt to cough or sneeze was peculiar and characteristic in the sound produced, in consequence of inability to close the glottis.

I made a note in this case of the absence of depression of the supraclavicular and intercostal spaces.

The patient had one or two attacks of hæmoptysis, but the most careful examination failed to detect any sign of an intra-thoracic tumour.

Under the influence of quinine and belladonna her symptoms were much relieved, but I regret to be unable to say what became of her eventually. In May, a note was made that she is unable to form a cough, but at that date her chief complaint was of her chronic rheumatism.

In the instance of a lady whom I saw but two or three times during her stay in London, there were extreme dyspnœa, very prolonged expiration and loss of voice, with dry cough, all of which symptoms improved after she had expectorated a complete cast of the trachea, reported to me as being seven inches long, and bifurcated at one end.

These brief observations may be of use in directing attention to the laryngeal and tracheal regions when investigating cases of presumed spasmodic asthma.

Another point to which I have often had my attention drawn by patients, has been the suddenness with which a paroxysm of breath difficulty seizes them. Patients lay a good deal of stress often on this symptom, and expect us to explain its cause.

So far as I have seen, these sudden paroxysms may occur in almost every form of dyspnœa.

Sudden paroxysmal dyspnœa is common

enough in laryngeal obstructions, also in tracheal stricture, *vide* Mackenzie's case in Path. Trans.; and in uncomplicated spasmodic asthma the attack sometimes comes on very suddenly, so that the patient has to leap from his bed and rush to the window.

In very chronic cases of fibroid phthisis and broncho-pneumonia equally sudden paroxysms often distress the patient. In cases of intra-thoracic aneurism or tumour sudden paroxysms of laryngeal dyspnœa are marked symptoms; and in many cases of valvular disease and cardiac dilatation patients complain of sudden dyspnœa, though the fits are not so spasmodic as they are when a tumour presses on some of the laryngeal nerves.

Though in most cases these very sudden paroxysms of dyspnœa are due to spasm of the glottis, yet, I have thought that at times a spasm of the diaphragm will cause a sudden attack of dyspnœa, for many patients with bronchitis and emphysema are liable to paroxysmal dyspnœa, while they refer the seat of their distress to the region of the diaphragm, rather than to that of

the larynx, the epigastrium being strongly
retracted, and sometimes the thoracic muscles
drawn into firm knots.

In some incurable cases of old degenerative
emphysema with stagnation of air in the chest,
no complaint is made of sudden dyspnœa, and
the movement of the diaphragm is very slight,
the muscle seeming almost to have lost power
of forcible contraction.

The two following cases, of no extraordinary
kind, will serve to illustrate the last made
remarks on the diaphragm.

CASE XVIII.—*Paroxysmal dyspnœa from diaphragmatic spasm.*

George S., æt. 60, has had cough and spitting
for ten years. Heart feeble, liver seems pushed
down by the emphysematous lungs. Chest is
extra resonant, and expiration very weak, except
at bases where it is rather coarse in character.

Complains much of sudden severe paroxysmal dyspnœa seizing him at night. Epigastrium drawn in ; muscles around rise up in
knots, with much sense of diaphragmatic stricture. Under iron and strychnine he improved
in a great degree.

CASE XIX.—*Example of tendency to diaphrag-*
matic paralysis.

Henry B., æt. 51, father died of asthma. Chest
very extra resonant, no sound of respiration, save
at bases.

Over larynx respiratory sound very feeble,
and the interchange of air in the chest seems
very imperfect. Dyspnœa constant, but not
paroxysmal at any time, no retraction of epigastrium, no diaphragmatic stricture, and very
little movement at this part of chest.

No improvement under a long course of treatment by iodide of potassium, strychnine and
various other medicines.

CHAPTER XI.

Hay asthma or summer catarrh.—Two forms of the disease.—
Researches of Dr. Pirrie—Treatment of hay asthma.—
Removal to the sea-coast.—Fumigations, inhalations, and
medicated snuffs.—Internal remedies.—Hay fever different
from hay asthma, and might well be called solar fever.—
It is a neurosis, but a paresis rather than a spasm.—Value
of tonics in treatment of solar fever.

IN this chapter a few remarks will be offered
on that form of specific asthma known as "hay
asthma," "hay fever," "summer catarrh," and
rarely and less appropriately as "summer bronchitis;" for it is in all its forms a disease with
which real bronchitis has nothing whatever to do,
since the wheezing and bronchial râles, that may,
in bad cases, be heard in the lungs, are due to
spasm and not to inflammation.

If this disease be known by a variety of names,
it has an infinitely greater number of drugs put
forth as curative agents; and while without

doubt many of these have at times marked curative efficacy, yet there is a great want of certainty in their action, and prescribing thus becomes a kind of hit or miss guesswork.

I consider we are mainly indebted to the researches of Dr. Pirrie for showing that there is a true spasmodic hay asthma, like any other form of spasmodic asthma, and probably due to the emanations of certain grasses affecting the mucous membrane of susceptible individuals. This form of the complaint recurs at intervals, and is promptly excited when the individual comes in contact with the aroma of a hay-field or a meadow of flowering grasses. The *nardus stricta* and *anthoxanthum odoratum* are the grasses whose emanations, set free by the sun's rays, cause this asthma. Some have thought that these grasses evolve benzoic acid, but I have never seen it proved to be this acid that excites hay asthma.

The symptoms are just those of spasmodic asthma, and there is often a running from the eyes and nose, irritation and sneezing, with mucous flux and catarrh.

From these catarrhal symptoms the disease obtains the name of "summer catarrh," and with a predominance sometimes of asthma, sometimes of catarrh, the complaint is apt to continue in an intermitting way during the summer-time, or as long as its specific exciting cause has chance of operation.

The most effective treatment is for the sufferer to remove from the neighbourhood of the source of his trouble, and he will be most out of harm's way probably on the sea-coast. If from any cause removal to the coast be impossible, then recourse must be had to remedial measures, and I regard local treatment of the mucous membrane as worthy of persevering trial.

Smoking tobacco in cigar or pipe is a well known source of relief to those who are liable to hay asthma. The practice should be to smoke as soon as ever the attack begins to threaten and at no other time, thus the full curative effect of the remedy is obtained.

As a simple means of local medication I have recently during the last summer recommended the use of Mr. Bird's inhaling pipe, the sponge being well soaked in spirit of camphor, to which some ether may be added. So far as present experience goes there is much comfort for those who are liable to hay asthma in the use of the pipe, and I expect it will become a remedy that will stand its ground well. Camphorated cigarettes, Slade's cigarettes, and the cigarettes de Joy may be trusted also as means of relief. When the flux is very troublesome and obstinate carbolic acid vapour or creasote inhalations from a Maw's or Nelson's inhaler may be used. If there be an aversion to a warm inhalation, then a solution of sulphate of zinc, or of alum with sulphate of iron, may be inhaled as spray from Clark's hand ball spray atomizer. The alum with the iron I place much confidence in as a tonic astringent. *See* Formulæ.

Bathing the nostrils and mouth with camphor julep is a useful practice just before going out in the heat of the sun. Helmholtz has drawn attention to the presence of vibrios in the mucous secretion of summer catarrh, and recommends the use locally of solution of quinine.

Cold water at 54? will dissolve sulphate of

quinine in the proportion of 1 in 740, and this solution may be used to the nasal passages by means of a spray atomizer, or of Mayer and Melzer's nasal douche.

I have tried iodine inhalations for the relief of summer catarrh, but have not found them of much use. Carbolic acid vapour from one of Savory and Moore's vaporizers is preferable to iodine, and far more convenient of employment.

Iodized camphor snuff, invented by Barrere, of Toulouse, is made by shaking together powdered camphor with one hundredth of iodine by weight, till the two bodies have combined into a brown powder. This may be carried in a small bottle, and a pinch occasionally taken by the nose; it causes at first some smarting, but from what experience I have as yet made with this snuff I feel encouraged to recommend it. Another snuff that I have for some time employed with advantage, is made by triturating 3 grains of iodide of sulphur with 2 drams of Pulv. glycyrrhizæ. This, like the iodized camphor, at first may cause transient irritation.

Of internal remedies one of the best I believe

to be Fowler's arsenical solution, taken in doses
of two to five drops three times a day in water.
Sulphate of iron, with or without sulphate of
quinine, is most valuable if there be much debility, and in a few cases iodide of potassium, or
else nitric acid seems to render real service. The
ethereal tincture of lobelia in full dose is reported
good as an anti-spasmodic medicine in hay
asthma, and the same has been said of dilute
hydrocyanic acid and aqua lauro-cerasi.

The complaint to which the name "hay fever"
is specially applicable differs in some respects from
the "hay asthma" that we have been describing,
and I have been able to recognise the distinction
before I knew how ably it had been pointed out
by Dr. Pirrie. True hay fever is a congestive
more than a spasmodic disease, and is apt to
attack the *habitués* of town when they go in the
heat of summer to the country; in some instances
it appears as a mere transient uneasiness, with
itching of the eyes and nose, some irritation of
the throat, and, perhaps, a little headache and
oppression at the chest. These slight symptoms
may vanish in a short time, or after the use of a
stimulant, and no more is thought of them.

In more thoroughly developed cases there is distinct fever of a somewhat remitting character, with now and then a tendency to shiver; there is also giddiness, heaviness of the head, with oppression at the chest and difficult respiration.

There may be catarrh, which appears due to a congested state of the mucous membrane, and at times mucous râle may be heard in the lungs.

This form of complaint seems due to solar heat, and I have thought it should be called summer fever or solar fever rather than hay fever, for I doubt if the smell of grass or hay has much to do with its causation, and I have known persons affected with this fever on arriving at the sea-side from London. The disease is tedious, very apt to recur, and not controlled so completely by change of air as true hay asthma is; neither do local applications appear to be of very marked service, though they may be tried in the forms already suggested, to palliate symptoms. The fact appears to be, just as Dr. Pirrie has said, that this affection is a paresis of the nervous centres. This I judge from the general symptoms, and from the fact that expectorant anti-bronchitic medicines are without effect on these symptoms, while tonics, and especially small doses of strychnine, as well as nux vomica, quinine, and sometimes arsenic, may be relied upon as useful and efficacious remedies.

The combination of saline aperients with tonics I believe to be here a good practice, as tending to relieve internal congestions, and so to cure and remove the congestive chills that distress and depress the patient at times.

Iodide of potassium and muriate of ammonia may be employed for this same purpose; and the former of these medicines, by relieving congestion of the mucous surface, I have known quickly to cut short troublesome catarrh.

Inasmuch as this hay fever is due to solar heat, and partakes in its nature somewhat of the character of sunstroke, it is necessary that the patient keep out of the sun, and the hot part of the day should be passed in a cool well-shaded apartment.

The diet should be on a generous scale, and with the meals a moderate allowance of dry sherry or weak brandy and water should be taken.

Cold salt water bathing is good as a means of strengthening the system generally, as well as of conquering that morbid nervous sensibility in which the essence of the malady consists.

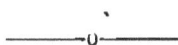

———o———

APPENDIX OF FORMULÆ.

FORMS FOR INHALATIONS TO BE USED COLD IN THE SPRAY ATOMIZER.—*See page* 156.

Sulphate of Zinc, 1 to 5 grains.

Alum, 5 to 10 grs.; Sulphate of Iron, 1 grain.

Tannin, 3 to 5 grains.

Liq. Ferri Perchloridi, ʒj. to ʒij..

Liq. Arsenicalis, 5 to 10 minims.

In each case to one ounce of distilled water.

FORM FOR USE IN THE INHALING PIPE.

See page 155.

Chloroform, ʒj.;

Tinct. Pyrethri, ʒij.;

Sp. Camphor., ʒv. M.

ʒj. to be used on the sponge of the pipe. (Mr. Bird.)

The inhalation of steam medicated with creasote, conium, iodine, &c., is best managed

M

with the Eclectic Inhaler of Dr. Mackenzie, which has the advantage of regulating and maintaining a proper temperature throughout the whole period of inhalation, as well as of rendering the process of inhaling easy and agreeable to the patient.

Another very excellent and efficient inhaler is the one known as Maw's double-valved inhaler, an improvement on the one invented by Nelson, inasmuch as it is provided with inspiratory and expiratory valves.

A third, that is very convenient and serviceable, is the inhaler invented some years ago by Curtis, of Baker Street.

INDEX.

London: M'GOWAN & CO., Steam Printers, Great Windmill Street, Haymarket, W.

* 9 7 8 3 7 4 2 8 2 6 8 9 3 *